SpringerBriefs in Electrical and Computer
Engineering

Naser Pour Aryan • Hans Kaim
Albrecht Rothermel

Stimulation and Recording Electrodes for Neural Prostheses

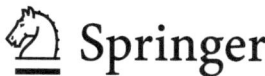

Springer

Naser Pour Aryan
Institute of Microelectronics
University of Ulm
Ulm, Germany

Hans Kaim
Institute of Microelectronics
University of Ulm
Ulm, Germany

Albrecht Rothermel
Institute of Microelectronics
University of Ulm
Ulm, Germany

ISSN 2191-8112   ISSN 2191-8120 (electronic)
ISBN 978-3-319-10051-7   ISBN 978-3-319-10052-4 (eBook)
DOI 10.1007/978-3-319-10052-4
Springer Cham Heidelberg New York Dordrecht London

Library of Congress Control Number: 2014948772

Printed on acid-free paper

Springer is part of Springer Science+Business Media (www.springer.com)

Preface

Neural diseases have always been a challenge to the humankind. Paralysis, blindness, and Parkinson's disease (PD) are examples. A biological treatment to many of these neurological dysfunctions is either not available or does not yet provide satisfactory results. Biomedical engineering provides an alternative to the biological cure. Together with neuroscience, engineering builds up a new concept in the field of practice, called neuroprosthetics. Neuroprosthetics pertains to the creation of neural prosthetics in order to eliminate sensory, motor, or cognitive malfunctions.

Treating these kinds of dysfunctions requires interfacing with patient's neural system. Depending on the application, electrical neural signals must be read or injected by the implant. This is accomplished through electrodes which connect the internal circuits of the device to tissue. The direction of the electrical signal defines the type of the electrode, which is thus classified as recording or stimulating. The electrical characteristics and the lifetime limitation of this component are very important in designing a neural prosthesis.

In this book we will address this major cornerstone of neuroprosthetics. Being part of a leading research group in the field of subretinal neurostimulators in Europe, we have gathered lots of knowledge through research and experiment, from which we will try to share the most interesting and relevant parts here. The attempt in this book is also to provide a general perspective to the matter, and not specifically from the point of view of visual stimulators.

The physiological aspects of neural stimulation and recording such as the necessary characteristics of the signals for successful stimulation or the features of the neural signals to be read by the prosthetic system are not the main topic of this essay, although sometimes mentioned as support for the discussions, and should be studied elsewhere.

This book is intended to avoid complicated theoretical discussions in the field of chemistry as far as possible. The writers are all from the engineering field and therefore the focus is put here on the practical aspect. The electrochemistry behind the subject is covered briefly. The concept and necessity of charge balance is investigated. The effect of electrode geometry on electrode lifetime is studied. Novel methods and hardware for electrode experimentation are developed and are introduced. Beside others, two kinds of electrode materials, titanium nitride and iridium, have been extensively investigated both qualitatively and quantitatively. The influence of the counter electrode on the safety margins and electrode lifetime in a two electrode system is explained. Electrode modeling is handled in the final chapter.

We would like to thank the people who helped us with the here accomplished research. We are thankful for the support provided by the following people: Steffen Kibbel, Mohammad Imam Hasan bin Asad, Anton Rommel, Jared Robertson, Sebastian Schleehauf, and Sandra Klinger. We are very thankful to Dr. Walter Wrobel for continuous interest and support.

Ulm, Germany   Naser Pour Aryan
July 2014   Hans Kaim
                                                                                                    Albrecht Rothermel

Contents

Acronyms

AIROF	Activated iridium oxide film
AWG	Arbitrary waveform generator
CPE	Constant phase element
CSC	Charge storage capacity
CV	Cyclic voltammetry
EIROF	Electrodeposited iridium oxide film
ESA	Electrochemical surface area
GSA	Geometric surface area
NHE	Normal hydrogen electrode
OCP	Open circuit potential
PBS	Phosphate buffered saline
PD	Parkinson's disease
SCE	Saturated calomel electrode
SHE	Standard hydrogen electrode
SIROF	Sputtered iridium oxide film
TiN	Titanium nitride
TIROF	Thermally prepared iridium oxide film

Authors

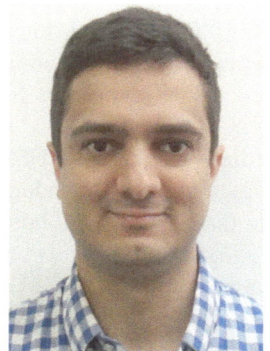

Naser Pour Aryan received his B.E. degree in electrical engineering from Ferdowsi University of Mashhad, Iran, in 2005 and M.Sc. degree in communication technology from the University of Ulm, Germany, in 2008. He received his Ph.D. degree from the University of Ulm in December 2013. He has been working as a researcher on the retinal prosthesis project at the University of Ulm since January 2008, studying and characterizing neural stimulation electrodes. He has had several publications on this topic.

Dr. Pour Aryan's research interests include mainly electrochemistry, analog and mixed signal circuits, modeling passive electrical structures, image processing, and optics.

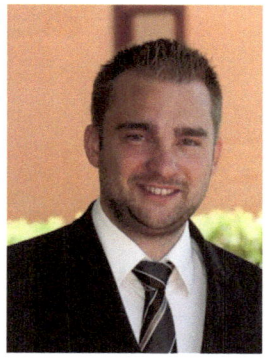

Hans Kaim received his Dipl.-Ing. degree in electrical engineering from the University of Ulm, Germany, in 2013. He has been working as a researcher on the retinal prosthesis project at the University of Ulm since January 2013, investigating and characterizing neural stimulation electrodes. His research interests include electrochemistry, modeling passive electrical structures, and analog and mixed signal circuits.

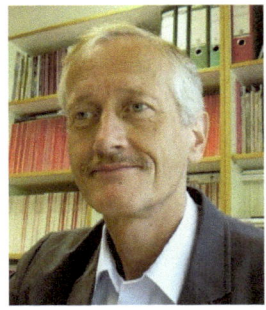 **Albrecht Rothermel** (M'90, SM'95) received his Dipl.-Ing. degree in electrical engineering from the University of Dortmund and Dr.-Ing. (Ph.D.) degree from the University of Duisburg, both Germany, in 1984 and 1989, respectively.

From 1985 to 1989, he was with the Fraunhofer Institute of Microelectronic Circuits and Systems, Duisburg, Germany, working on integrated digital CMOS and BiCMOS circuits for high-speed applications. From 1990 to 1993, he was with Thomson Consumer Electronics (Thomson multimedia), Corporate Research, Villingen-Schwenningen, Germany. He worked on digital signal processing concepts for present and future TV and HDTV sets. Then as Manager of the IC design laboratory, he was involved in analog and mixed circuit design for audio and video.

Since 1994, he has been with the Institute of Microelectronics, University of Ulm, Germany, as a Professor of Electrical Engineering. His research interests include analog and mixed signal circuits for various applications including implantable sensors and stimulators, and digital signal processing algorithms for video applications, mostly in automotive environments.

Dr. Rothermel was a guest scientist at Thomson Multimedia in Indianapolis, USA (1997), at the Edith-Cowan University in Perth, WA (2003), and at the Shandong University in Jinan, China (2006). He has published more than 130 papers, book chapters, and patents. He received the 1985 outstanding young scientist award of the German VDE, the 1991 outstanding publication award of the German GME, the 2003 award for remarkable cooperation between industry and university, and the 2006 best paper award of the IEEE ICCE. After acting as associate editor of the IEEE JSSC, TPC-Chair of the IEEE ICCE-B, and distinguished lecturer of the IEEE, he now is a member of the program committees of ESSCIRC and ICCE.

He is member of the German Society of Electrical Engineers (VDE), the German TV and Cinema Technology Society (FKTG), and senior member of the IEEE.

Chapter 1
Stimulation and Recording Electrodes: General Concepts

In prosthetic devices, electrodes are the interfaces between the implant system and the body. Electrodes may be used for neural stimulation or neural signal recording according to the application. The signals to be recorded are typically small, i.e. some tens of microvolts for single pulse activity to a maximum amplitude of around 80 mV for intracellular potentials measured for example by fine-tipped electrolyte-filled glass micropipettes in cognitive studies in brain machine interface. On the opposite, neural stimulation sometimes needs relatively high electrode voltages and current densities, sometimes as high as several volts, so it may lead to a high enough energy transfer triggering chemical reactions that involve corrosion and changes in electrode properties.

The electrodes used in neuroprosthetics appear in different sizes and areas. Regarding area, one could categorize electrodes into microelectrodes and macro-electrodes. Although there is not a clear boundary, an area lower than $10,000\,\mu m^2$ corresponds to a microelectrode and above $100,000\,\mu m^2$ ($0.001\,cm^2$) to a macro-electrode [1]. Macroelectrodes are sometimes much larger, such as deep brain stimulation electrodes with an area of $0.06\,cm^2$. Electrodes come in different shapes. Some electrodes used are flat and disk or square shaped, like the ones used in visual prostheses, and some like the ones used in cognitive control of prosthetic limbs for paralyzed patients have the shape of a shaft. The electrode of cardiac pacemaker is helical (Fig. 1.1).

Except for the case of the micropipette electrode for which the conducting electrode material is an electrolyte, the electrodes are built from metals or conducting ceramics like titanium nitride (TiN). Therefore, the boundary between the electrode and the electrolyte forms a phase boundary. For a well conducting electrolyte, this phase boundary can be modeled by a capacitance whose dielectric consists of two consecutive water molecule layers. The conducting plates of this capacitor are the electrode and the electrolyte. The two layers are the water dipoles adsorbed on the electrode surface and the hydration envelope of the ions in the vicinity of the

© The Author(s) 2015
N. Pour Aryan et al., *Stimulation and Recording Electrodes for Neural Prostheses*,
SpringerBriefs in Electrical and Computer Engineering 78,
DOI 10.1007/978-3-319-10052-4_1

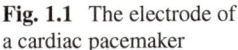

Fig. 1.1 The electrode of a cardiac pacemaker

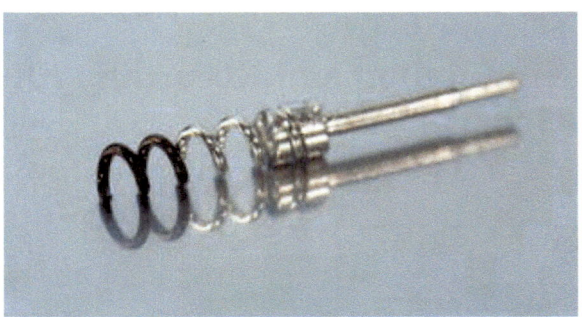

electrode-electrolyte phase boundary. This capacitor is called Helmholtz double layer capacitor. In practice, especially when the electrolyte has a low concentration and therefore a high resistance, another capacitance in series with the Helmholtz double layer is considered, the so called Gouy-Chapman capacitance. It corresponds to a diffuse area of space charge which neutralizes the immobilized charge directly on the electrode surface. This capacitor is neglected in the following.

Charge injection into the electrode may be through charging and discharging the Helmholtz capacitor. When this capacitor is charged, positive and negative charges (in solid electrode, electrons and ions; in solution, only ions) gather on its two plates, namely the electrode and the electrolyte. The electrode is said to be polarized. Metal and many ceramic electrodes are said to be polarizable, because the interface between their surface and the electrolyte can be regarded as a chargeable capacitor. The micropipette electrode mentioned above is non-polarizable. There is no phase boundary here and thus no interface capacitor can exist. The charge transfer is done by ions flowing into or out of the solution from the electrode body.

Depending on the material and especially at higher charge magnitudes, charge transfer can occur by electron transfer across the surface. This happens through redox reactions at the electrode surface. For example, the anions are oxidized and transformed into gas at anode (e.g. Cl^- into Cl_2) and the cations are reduced and precipitate on cathode (e.g. Cu^{2+} into Cu). If a considerable amount of electron transfer (ideally unlimited) occurs at already low electrode-electrolyte potential differences, the charges can not be separated across the phase boundary and no capacitor can exist. The material is again non-polarizable, even if there is a phase boundary. One example is the silver-silver chloride electrode which is used as a reference electrode and can be considered as ideally non-polarizable for low current magnitudes (this electrode will be explained below). In practice the electrodes lie somewhere between being perfectly polarizable or perfectly non-polarizable.

If the material is polarizable, like metals or TiN, for lower charge injection densities, capacitive currents flow into the tissue or the solution representing the tissue. Here only the electrode Helmholtz capacitance is charged to make current injection possible. Higher charge injections require a charge transfer across the electrode surface through the redox reactions.

When producing electrodes for neural stimulation within the body, choosing the best electrode material for the application is important. Several criteria must be considered when choosing these materials. Materials that consume very little power while still operating efficiently and safely are ideal. It is also important for the electrodes to be as small as possible so the implanted chip can maximize performance while minimizing intrusion to the patient [6].

Tow types of area are considered for the electrodes: real surface area and geometric surface area. Geometric surface area is the traditional idea of surface area (length × width for a rectangular electrode, $\pi \times (\text{radius})^2$ for a circular electrode, etc.). In practice, if the electrode surface is rough or porous, the area at which the electrode and electrolyte touch is much larger than the geometric surface area. This interface area is called real surface area. Real surface area (or electrochemical surface area) factors in the surface roughness of the electrode being used and can be orders of magnitude larger than the geometric surface area. A rough electrode has a higher Helmholtz capacitance compared to a smooth surface. In the case of faradaic current flow, more surface chemical reactions can occur on a rough electrode than a smooth one with the same geometric surface area. The real surface area is usually described with a surface roughness factor (the ratio of real surface area to geometric surface area) which can sometimes be higher than 2,000 [5]. Figure 1.2 helps to show the difference between the real surface area and the geometric surface area. Table 1.1 lists typical roughness factor ranges for common types of stimulating electrodes used in cardiac pacemakers.

Fractal TiN, with a high electrochemical surface area, is applied extensively as coating for cardiac pacing electrodes, mainly because the electrode polarization during a pacing pulse is minimal [1]. However, under the high rate, high current

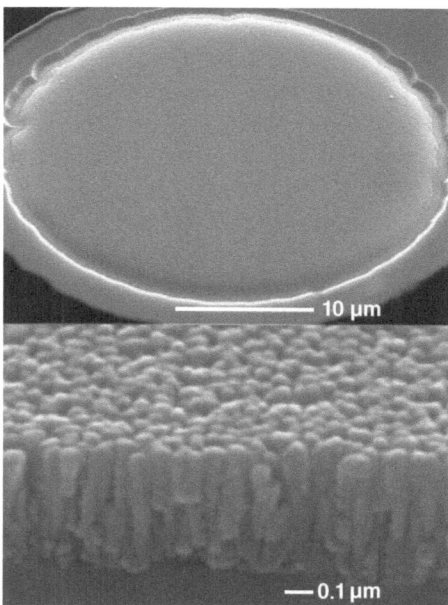

Fig. 1.2 The porous (fractal) surface of TiN electrode enlarges the surface area; the fractal structure is visible at the *bottom*. The picture is from Multi Channel Systems GmbH, with permission

Table 1.1 Typical roughness factor ranges for common cardiac stimulation electrodes [5]

Material	Type	Roughness factor
Titanium nitride	Microporous	>400
Titanium nitride	Fractal	>2,000
Iridium	Fractal	>1,000

Fig. 1.3 View of a pore profile illustrating the pore resistance (R1...R3) and double-layer capacitance (C1...C3) elements that make up a delay-line and time-constant for accessing all the ESA and its associated double-layer capacity, picture adapted from [1]

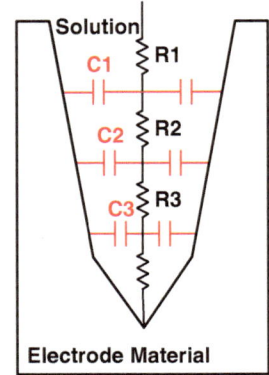

density conditions of a neural stimulation pulse, access to all the available charge is limited by pore resistance [1]. The amount of the charge injected by a material before unwanted redox reactions occur is called charge injection capacity. A higher real surface area increases the double layer capacitance of the electrode. Therefore, the electrode-electrolyte capacitance voltage is smaller for the same amount of injected charge. This avoids occurrence of unwanted redox reactions, as they preferably occur at higher electrode-electrolyte interface voltage drops. For all porous electrodes, pore resistance exerts a geometric limitation on the increase in charge injection capacity that can be attained by increasing the "electrochemical surface area (ESA)"/"geometric surface area (GSA)" ratio. A schematic view of a pore and electrolyte in a porous electrode coating is illustrated in Fig. 1.3. The solution resistance and capacitance on the inner surface of the pore form a delay-line with a time-constant dependent on the pore geometry, electrolyte resistivity, and the interface double-layer capacitance. The result is that the total ESA of the electrode is not accessed at the current densities encountered during current and voltage edges. Narrower and deeper pores result in higher time-constants, and their charge-injection capacity is more difficult to access than that of electrodes with shallow pores. Both TiN and iridium oxide have higher measurable electrode-electrolyte capacitance per unit area with 0.5 ms pulses compared to 0.2 ms [6], because more real electrode area is accessible in lower frequencies and the diffusion rates of the charge carriers in the solution are limited.

The surface roughness factor is experimentally determined by measuring the amount of chemicals that can be adsorbed onto the surface of the electrode [3]. As the porosity of an electrode increases, the real surface area increases and the surface impedance decreases. The real surface area of a porous electrode also increases when the thickness of the porous metal increases.

Another method to estimate the real surface area in materials like TiN which inject charge capacitively is cyclic voltammetry. Due to the intrinsic delays present in the topography of electrode surface structures (pores RC delays) explained above, the large interface capacitance of TiN measured with slow cyclic voltammetry is not available at fast rates of current injection [4].

Lower electrode impedances are favorable for both stimulating and recording electrodes. A certain amount of current density is required to initiate stimulation. A high electrode impedance will therefore mean high electrode voltages for a given current density which result in electrochemical reactions which may damage both the electrode and the tissue. In recording electrodes, the signals to be recorded are very small, in the order of millivolts to microvolts. The signal may be lost in the noisy ionic environment if the electrode impedance is not low enough [2]. Larger electrodes are preferred as the total resistance of the solution in the vicinity of the electrode there is smaller and therefore the thermal noise due to the resistance in series with the electrode double layer capacitance is decreased.

For extracellular signal recording, as the signal itself has almost no DC and contains frequencies between hundreds and thousands of Hertz, the electrode must feature a large interface capacitance, otherwise the electrode impedance is too high for this low frequency range. More porous electrodes are favorable.

Recording electrodes should be used in an input voltage amplitude range where they are linear, otherwise the nonlinearity would deform the shape of the recorded signal. In Chap. 5 it will be explained how to determine the linearity range of an electrode using a method called impedance spectroscopy.

1.1 Cyclic Voltammetry and Impedance Spectroscopy

Cyclic voltammetry (CV) uncovers a lot about the nature of charge transfer at the electrode surface. The standard measurement setup has three electrodes. The voltage of the working electrode (the electrode under test, here the stimulation or the recording electrode) is varied against a reference electrode. The reference electrode is used as a potential reference and sets the solution potential to a definite value. The result is a ramp voltage on the working electrode. The third electrode, the counter electrode, is used to close the circuit, i.e. ideally no current flows into the reference electrode. The current flowing from the working into the counter electrodes is measured. After a certain voltage limit is reached, the voltage is decreased till another lower limit is reached. This process may be repeated (i.e. the potential is cyclically varied). A cyclic voltammogram is the resulting current versus voltage difference measurement trace. The peaks in the graph correspond to different redox reactions. Also in case of purely capacitive charge injection, the amount of double layer capacitance can be assessed from the cyclic voltammogram. An example for cyclic voltammetry is shown for iridium oxide and TiN in Fig. 6.1.

The reference electrode is a very important component in CV. When a polarizable material like a metal is immersed in a solution, an electrode potential builds up at the electrode-electrolyte phase boundary at the thermodynamic equilibrium. This potential is due to the oxidation of the metal atoms as they turn into positive ions and enter the solution and the reduction of the ions as they are adsorbed on the metal surface. For example if a Zn electrode is immersed into $ZnSO_4$ solution, Zn atoms begin to solve in very small magnitudes into the solution and form Zn^{2+} ions:

$$Zn(s) \leftrightarrow Zn^{2+}(aq) + 2e^- \tag{1.1}$$

The resulting electrons remain on the electrode. So a potential difference develops at the interface which is approximately 1 V.

Unfortunately it is not possible to measure this electrode potential in practice; therefore, the so called reference electrodes are used which feature a stable electrode potential. The reference electrode must be kept thermodynamically in equilibrium, i.e. very little or ideally no current must flow into it, otherwise the electrode potential deviates from what is expected from the equilibrium state. There are different kinds of reference electrodes like the standard hydrogen electrode and the silver-silver chloride (Ag|AgCl) electrode. Silver-silver chloride electrode is the most prevalent in the physiological studies and is shown in Fig. 1.4.

In order to achieve a defined electrode-electrolyte potential difference (electrode potential), a solution with a defined concentration is contained inside a plastic or glass tube. The solution is usually chosen as a saturated chloride solution, e.g. KCl. In order to avoid the reference electrode from changing the main electrolyte environment, a limited electrolyte connection is available between the KCl solution and the main electrolyte through a porous plug or diaphragm at the electrode tip which is permeable for chloride ions. The corresponding reduction reaction is:

$$AgCl(s) + e^- \leftrightarrow Ag(s) + Cl^- \quad E^0 = +0.23\,V$$

$E^0 = +0.23\,V$ is called the standard reduction potential which is measured against another reference electrode, the standard hydrogen electrode (SHE) which has by definition an electrode potential of zero. This definition is necessary as the electrode potential cannot be experimentally measured in practice. As the chloride solution is saturated (above 3.5 mol/kg concentration) and thus the concentration is not unity as in the standard condition, the saturated silver-silver chloride electrode has a potential of $+0.197\,V$ against SHE.

In some literature, instead of using a saturated chloride solution, another definite concentration is considered. With a 3 and 1 molal (mol/kg) KCL solution, the electrode potential is $+0.21\,V$ and $+0.235\,V$ versus SHE, respectively.

Fig. 1.4 Saturated Ag-AgCl
reference electrode

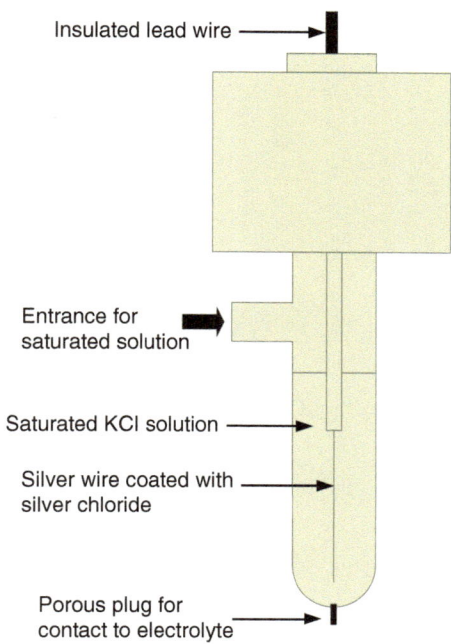

Insulated lead wire

Entrance for
saturated solution

Saturated KCl solution

Silver wire coated with
silver chloride

Porous plug for
contact to electrolyte

Due to the glass tube, the silver-silver chloride electrode can be put in the same solution vessel containing also the working and counter electrodes as shown in Fig. 1.5. If a reference electrode does not have this containing tube, it must be dipped in a separate solution vessel. This vessel is then electrically connected to the vessel containing the two other electrodes through a salt bridge.

The application of silver-silver chloride electrode is limited to outside the body, e.g. skin electrodes for ECG or EEG recording. In this case they are made wet by a chloride ion containing fluid or paste.

In order to perform CV a potentiostat is used. The basic three electrode potentiostat setup is shown in Fig. 1.5. V_{IN} is the input voltage from the potentiostat. As the reference electrode has a definite electrode potential, it is used to set the potential of the electrolyte. The counter electrode does not affect the solution potential and only carries current through redox reactions which are actually not a point of interest in CV. So carrying current and setting the solution potential are done by different electrodes.

The three electrode system eliminates the dependence of the measured current on the counter electrode. If the amplifier has a very high amplification and zero input bias current, it can be shown that in the equivalent electrical circuit of the

Fig. 1.5 Three-electrode
electrochemical cell

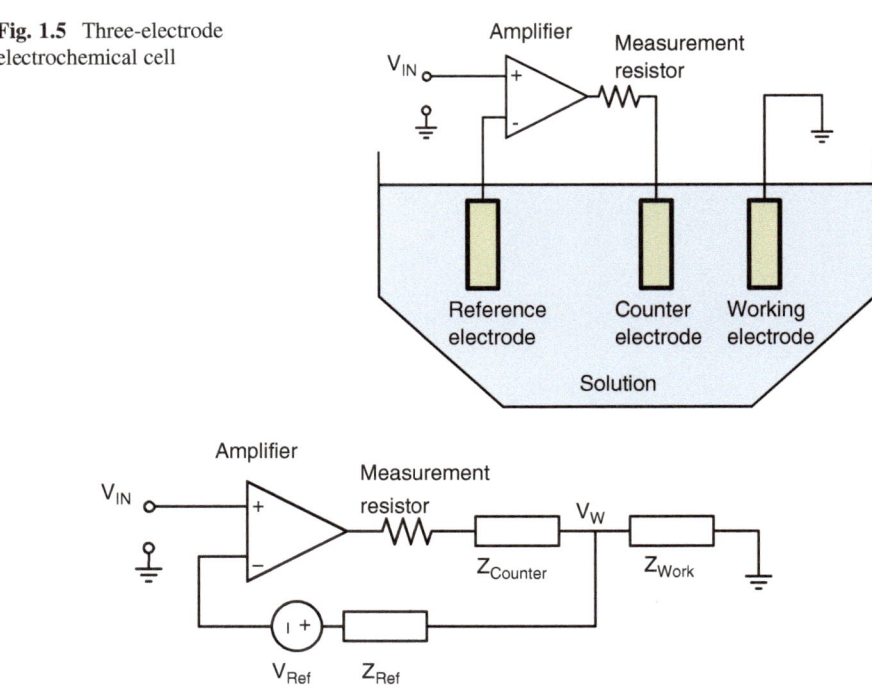

Fig. 1.6 The equivalent circuit of the three-electrode electrochemical cell

three cell setup shown in Fig. 1.6, $V_{IN} = V_W + V_{Ref}$. The current flowing into the working electrode is measured through the measurement resistor. The effect of the impedance of the counter electrode on the measured current is eliminated.

The same setup is used in impedance spectroscopy. Here, electrode impedance composed of amplitude and phase is measured by putting a sine voltage with varying frequency (V_{IN} in Fig. 1.6) on the electrode (a DC offset of V_{Ref} will exist at V_W) and measuring the resulting current amplitude and phase shift over the frequency. The impedance spectrum of the electrode under test, i.e. Z_{Work} versus frequency of V_{IN}, is determined. An electrode model can be extracted from the resulting impedance data. It is usually composed of the prevalent linear components in electrical engineering like resistor and capacitor and components which are defined for the especial use in electrochemistry. One of these elements is introduced in Chap. 8, namely the constant phase element.

For monopolar stimulation arrangement with small microelectrode and a large distant counter electrode a two electrode system can be used for impedance spectroscopy. This will be investigated in Chap. 5.

References

1. Cogan SF (2008) Neural stimulation and recording electrodes. Tech. rep., EIC Laboratories
2. Franks W, Schenker I, Schmutz P, Hierlemann A (2005) Impedance characterization and modeling of electrodes for biomedical applications. Biomedical Engineering, IEEE Transactions on 52(7):1295–1302, DOI 10.1109/TBME.2005.847523
3. McCreery D (2004) The Problem of Safe and Effective Stimulation of Neural Tissue. World Scientific
4. Patan M, Shah T, Sahin M (2006) Charge injection capacity of TiN electrodes for an extended voltage range. Conf Proc IEEE Eng Med Biol Soc 1:890–2, URL http://www.biomedsearch.com/nih/Charge-injection-capacity-TiN-electrodes/17946870.html
5. Stieglitz T (2004) Materials for stimulation and recording. Tech. rep., Neural Prosthetics Group, Fraunhofer Institute for Biomedical Engineering
6. Weiland JD, Anderson DJ, Humayun MS (2002) In vitro electrical properties for iridium oxide versus titanium nitride stimulating electrodes. Biomedical Engineering, IEEE Transactions on 49(12):1574–1579, DOI 10.1109/TBME.2002.805487

Chapter 2
Irreversible and Reversible Redox Reactions: Water Window

As mentioned above, capacitive charging cannot deliver enough current if current density exceeds certain limits. The potential difference between the active (working) and the counter electrodes (used to close the electrical circuit) must remain low enough so that (almost) no redox reactions occur, if only capacitive charge injection is to follow.

Although absence of any redox reactions is ideal for electrode lifetime, these reactions are very hard to avoid. As soon as the electrode materials come in contact with an ionic solution, lots of different reactions may occur, even if no current flows into the electrode. Consider a piece of iron immersed in saline solution. After enough time, rust appears on the iron surface. Corrosion occurs following simultaneous reduction and oxidation reactions on the surface. While the metal is oxidized, oxygen (O_2) or H^+ ions are reduced at the same time to complete the redox reaction.

Corrosion is not limited to relatively reactive materials like iron. In TiN, in spite of the rather capacitive nature of the metal-electrode interface for charge injection, corrosion occurs at zero electrode potential in distilled water. However, the reaction is very slow and practically does not result in considerable damage even after long periods of time [6]. Titanyl (TiO_2^{2+}) ions are produced:

$$2TiN + 4H_2O \rightarrow 2TiO_2^{2+} + N_2 + 8H^+ + 12e^- \qquad (2.1)$$

When no current flows into the electrode, the anodic current due to all the oxidation reactions and the cathodic current due to all the reduction reactions are equal. The value of this current is called the corrosion current. It is difficult but possible to experimentally measure this current indirectly for a special material in contact with some electrolyte.[1]

---

[1] For details on this please refer to the corresponding application notes on www.gamry.com.

© The Author(s) 2015
N. Pour Aryan et al., *Stimulation and Recording Electrodes for Neural Prostheses*,
SpringerBriefs in Electrical and Computer Engineering 78,
DOI 10.1007/978-3-319-10052-4_2

Other redox reactions become thermodynamically favorable at higher electrode potentials. It is practically impossible to find a limit where no redox reaction occurs at all. For example if iridium or iridium oxide comes in contact with water with acidic environment, the following half reactions are possible.

$$Ir_2O_3(s) + 6H^+(aq) + 6e^- \leftrightarrow 2Ir(s) + 3H_2O \qquad E^0 = +0.926 \text{ V}$$

$$IrO_2(s) + 4H^+(aq) + 4e^- \leftrightarrow Ir(s) + 2H_2O \qquad E^0 = +0.926 \text{ V}$$

$$2IrO_2(s) + 2H^+(aq) + 2e^- \leftrightarrow Ir_2O_3(s) + H_2O \qquad E^0 = +0.926 \text{ V}$$

$$IrO_2(s) + 4H^+(aq) + e^- \leftrightarrow Ir^{3+}(aq) + 2H_2O \qquad E^0 = +0.233 \text{ V}$$

$$Ir^{3+}(aq) + 3e^- \leftrightarrow Ir(s) \qquad E^0 = +1.156 \text{ V}$$

The corresponding standard reduction potentials (E^0) are given. The potentials were measured with a standard hydrogen electrode (SHE) as reference. Reduction potential is a measure of the tendency of a material to acquire electrons and be thereby reduced. Standard conditions are the conditions in which the solutes are at an effective concentration (activity) of 1 mol/dm^3 and gases are at a partial pressure of 1 bar. Temperature is 25 °C and pH $= 7$.[2] The standard reduction potentials of the above half-reactions are different. Therefore, avoiding every half-reaction requires obeying a different voltage limit. The above potential values cannot be used directly in practice (for neural electrode stimulation studies) as the reference electrode is not SHE here. However, the differences are helpful. Every redox reaction is composed of a simultaneous reduction and oxidation. These two have distinct E^0 values. The difference between these two determines whether the reaction is theoretically spontaneous if a certain working versus counter electrode potential difference exists. In practice, effects called collectively as overpotential affect this spontaneity. Overpotential means that a higher potential is necessary to ignite the redox reaction than anticipated from the reduction potential values. It has different reasons like the activation energy of the redox reactions occurring at the electrode surface.

As avoiding all the redox reactions is not possible, other limits for reliable electrode operation are necessary. This can be settled knowing that not all reactions damage the electrodes. The reactions in which the products are immobilized on the electrode surface may be reversed if the electrode current direction is reversed. These are called reversible reactions [8]. Two examples are:

$$Pt + H_2O \leftrightarrow PtO + 2H^+ + 2e^-$$

$$Ir + 2H_2O \leftrightarrow Ir(OH)_2 + 2H^+ + 2e^-$$

---

[2]In contrast to electrochemistry where pH $= 0$ at standard conditions, in biochemistry pH $= 7$ holds.

These processes do not damage the electrodes if charge injection balance into the electrode is guaranteed. Charge balance roughly means that the total amount of charge injected into the electrode remains zero. This will be explained in detail in the next chapter.

Another group of reactions are the irreversible reactions. These are reactions for which the products are not immobilized on the metal surface. This is the case when gases are produced or when the products spread into the solution by diffusion processes. Irreversible reactions cause corrosion of electrode materials [8]. An example is:

$$Pt + 4Cl^- \rightarrow [PtCl_4]^{2-} + 2e^-$$

As platinum and gold have similar chemical properties (neighbors in the periodic table of elements and both belonging to the group of transition metals) and the complexes $[PtCl_4]^{2-}$ and $[AuCl_4]^{2-}$ have similar chemical structures, gold dissolution in a medium containing chloride ions (like phosphate buffered saline[3] and body environment) is also irreversible:

$$Au + 4Cl^- \rightarrow [AuCl_4]^- + 3e^-$$

This is probably the reason why gold electrodes suffer dissolution into the tissue environment. Alan Chow et al. [3] have shown that the use of gold as electrode material in visual prosthetics is inappropriate due to gold electrode dissolution into the body environment. Furthermore it was shown that a lack of electrical activity avoids gold dissolution. In the current study gold dissolution on the structures containing gold was observed after symmetric voltages of ± 2 V was applied for 24 h.

Another important irreversible reaction is the hydrolysis of water [8]. The two half reactions occurring on separate electrodes (cathode and anode) are:

$$2H_2O + 2e^- \rightarrow H_2 \uparrow +2OH^-$$

$$2H_2O \rightarrow O_2 \uparrow +4H^+ + 4e^-$$

These reactions cannot be reversed once they occur, because the product escapes the surface immediately. In order to prevent electrolysis, the voltage waveform on the electrode interface capacitance is required to never exceed the so called water window limits [4]. Water window is different for different electrode materials [4]. Measured with silver-silver chloride as the reference electrode, water window is between -0.6 and $+0.8$ V for iridium oxide electrodes [10] and ± 0.9 V for TiN [4].

---

[3]One liter of phosphate buffered saline (PBS) contains 8 g NaCl, 0.2 g KCl, 1.44 g Na_2HPO_4, 0.24 g KH_2PO_4. HCl is used to adjust the pH to 7.4 [1].

Fig. 2.1 (**a**) Working versus
counter electrode model.
(**b**) Working electrode model

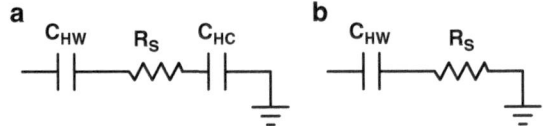

For electrochemical safety, the transients of the electrode-electrolyte interface
voltage must stay inside the water window even for pulse widths as short as
0.1–0.5 ms [5, 7, 9–11]. For shorter pulse widths this is even more critical, because
with shorter pulses, the reversible reactions cannot be fully utilized, as the reactions
don't have an unlimited speed. Therefore, for shorter pulses, the charge available
from reversible processes is smaller [7].

The reversibility of the reactions supports the electrode lifetime only if they
are fast enough. The relatively low safe charge injection limit of iridium oxide
electrodes used in [5] was due to either slow redox kinetics of that type of iridium
oxide or diffusion limitations. The pulses used were 0.5 ms long. To find out
the charge injection, the electrode voltages were kept inside the safe potential
range. Cyclic voltammograms with scan rates as high as 200 mV/s showed that the
reactions on the TiN electrodes are not wholly reversible [2].

Both the working and the counter electrodes have a double layer capacitance
and the solution in between exhibits a resistance called spreading resistance R_S.
The working versus counter electrode pair have a model illustrated in Fig. 2.1a.
C_{HW} and C_{HC} are the double layer capacitors of the working and the counter
electrodes, respectively. In monopolar stimulation structure in which the counter
electrode is much larger than the working microelectrode and is far away, the
voltage drop on the counter electrode phase boundary is usually negligible and the
large double layer capacitance C_{HC} of the counter electrode can be neglected in
the model. The resulting model for the working electrode is the one in Fig. 2.1b.
From here on, the impedance of the counter electrode is neglected in the discussions.

In theory, as explained above, in order to determine the charge injection capacity
of an electrode the voltage on the Helmholtz capacitance must be monitored.
Therefore, in literature the voltage drop on the spreading resistance is usually
subtracted from the electrode potential to achieve the voltage drop on the Helmholtz
capacitance [7, 9]. However, as is discussed in Chap. 4, this may sometimes lead to
too liberal charge injection boundaries.

The voltage drop on the electrolyte is equal to $= I \times R_S$, and is called access
voltage. Here I is the injected current into the solution and R_S is the electrolyte's
spreading resistance. Figure 2.2 illustrates an example for phase boundary voltage
extraction. In the figure, i.p.p. is the interpulse potential, E_c is the maximum
cathodic potential, and E_a is the maximum anodic potential both after access
voltage correction. The electrode was a smooth disk with a diameter of 1.1 mm
(macroelectrode) cut from a platinum foil and mounted in a silicone rubber support.

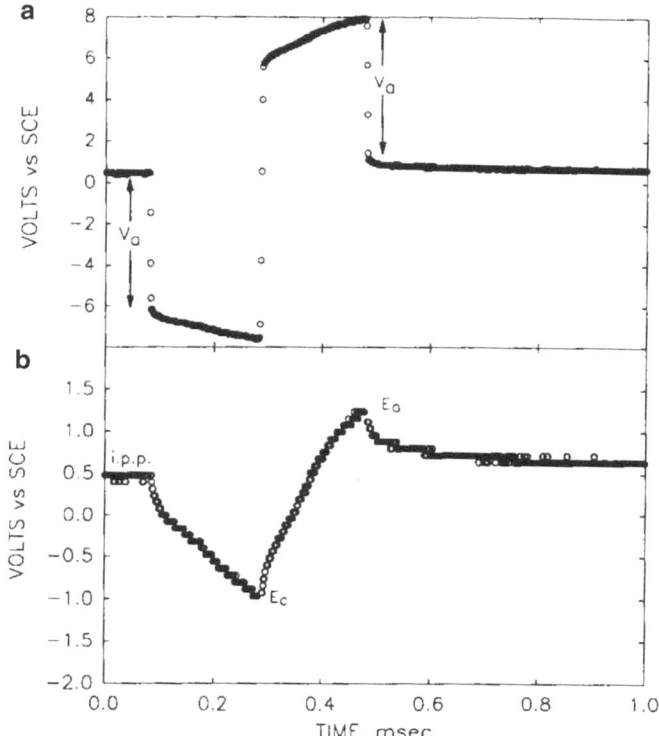

Fig. 2.2 (**a**) Directly measured electrode potential. (**b**) Same waveform plotted on expanded scale after correction for access voltage V_a (by subtracting V_a), this waveform should be kept inside the water window (−0.6 to +0.9 V for platinum) for safe operation. The pulse length and the charge injection density were 0.2 ms and 400 $\mu C/cm^2$, respectively. Biphasic cathodic first symmetrical current pulses were used. A saturated calomel electrode (SCE) was used as the reference electrode. From [7], with permission ©1990 IEEE

References

1. (August 2010) http://protocolsonline.com/
2. Bellanger G, Rameau JJ (1995) Corrosion of titanium nitride deposits on AISI 630 stainless steel used in radioactive water with and without chloride at pH 11. Electrochimica Acta 40(15):2519–2532, DOI 10.1016/0013-4686(94)00326-V, URL http://www.sciencedirect.com/science/article/pii/001346869400326V
3. Chow AY, Pardue MT, Chow VY, Peyman GA, Liang C, Perlman JI, Peachey NS (2001) Implantation of silicon chip microphotodiode arrays into the cat subretinal space. Neural Systems and Rehabilitation Engineering, IEEE Transactions on 9(1):86–95, DOI 10.1109/7333.918281
4. Cogan SF (2008) Neural stimulation and recording electrodes. Tech. rep., EIC Laboratories
5. Janders M, Egert U, Stelzle M, Nisch W (1996) Novel thin film titanium nitride micro-electrodes with excellent charge transfer capability for cell stimulation and sensing applications. In: Engineering in Medicine and Biology Society, 1996. Bridging Disciplines for Biomedicine. Proceedings of the 18th Annual International Conference of the IEEE, vol 1, pp 245–247 vol. 1, DOI 10.1109/IEMBS.1996.656936

6. Lavrenko VA, Shvets VA, Makarenko GN (2001) Comparative study of the chemical resistance of titanium nitride and stainless steel in media of the oral cavity. Powder Metallurgy and Metal Ceramics 40:630–636, URL http://dx.doi.org/10.1023/A:1015296323497, 10.1023/A:1015296323497

7. Rose TL, Robblee LS (1990) Electrical stimulation with Pt electrodes. VIII. Electrochemically safe charge injection limits with 0.2 ms pulses (neuronal application). Biomedical Engineering, IEEE Transactions on 37(11):1118–1120, DOI 10.1109/10.61038

8. Stieglitz T (2004) Materials for stimulation and recording. Tech. rep., Neural Prosthetics Group, Fraunhofer Institute for Biomedical Engineering

9. Terasawa Y, Tashiro H, Uehara A, Saitoh T, Ozawa M, Tokuda T, Ohta J (2006) The development of a multichannel electrode array for retinal prostheses. Journal of Artificial Organs 9:263–266, URL http://dx.doi.org/10.1007/s10047-006-0352-1, 10.1007/s10047-006-0352-1

10. Weiland JD, Anderson DJ, Humayun MS (2002) In vitro electrical properties for iridium oxide versus titanium nitride stimulating electrodes. Biomedical Engineering, IEEE Transactions on 49(12):1574–1579, DOI 10.1109/TBME.2002.805487

11. Zhou DM, Greenberg RJ (2003) Electrochemical characterization of titanium nitride microelectrode arrays for charge-injection applications. In: Engineering in Medicine and Biology Society, 2003. Proceedings of the 25th Annual International Conference of the IEEE, vol 2, pp 1964–1967 Vol. 2, DOI 10.1109/IEMBS.2003.1279831

Chapter 3
Charge Balance and Safe Operation Conditions

In order to ensure long electrode lifetime, charge balance is necessary for electrostimulation. If charge balance is obeyed, the reversible reactions are used to prevent the electrode state to change over time. In the literature, it is usually assumed that when biphasic, charge-balanced current pulses are used, ideal charge balance is achieved. Figure 3.1 shows three common types of biphasic charge balanced current pulses mentioned in the literature. The monophasic capacitor-coupled waveform is generated through a capacitor discharge circuit [1].

Although the above statement is right when the simple model of Fig. 2.1b is assumed for the electrode, it is not precise in the general case.

It is stated in [3] that even completely symmetrical bi-phasic current waveforms would not result in charge balance and will cause a residual voltage and charge build-up on the electrodes. The reason is the presence of a faradaic resistor R_{FW} parallel to the electrode-electrolyte interface capacitor. This resistor models the electron transfer across the electrode-electrolyte surface. The resulting electrode model which is called Randles model is shown in Fig. 3.2. For example in [3], for sputtered iridium oxide electrodes with $400\,\mu$m diameter in saline solution, $R_{FW} = 17.12\,\text{k}\Omega$, $R_S = 2.1\,\text{k}\Omega$ and $C_{HW} = 909\,\text{nF}$ were extracted using the step response of the electrode voltage to an input current.

The R_{FW} resistance value depends on the electrode-electrolyte voltage drop as more redox reactions occur at higher voltage magnitudes and thus more electrons are transferred. Therefore, the higher this voltage the lower the resistance value.

Considering the Randles model, an accurate definition of ideal charge balance is that the net current flowing into R_{FW} is zero over time. If this average be zero, under the assumption that only reversible reactions are present, all the reactions are completely reversed and the electrode material status remains unchanged. This condition is not achieved completely by biphasic symmetrical current pulses into the electrode.

© The Author(s) 2015
N. Pour Aryan et al., *Stimulation and Recording Electrodes for Neural Prostheses*,
SpringerBriefs in Electrical and Computer Engineering 78,
DOI 10.1007/978-3-319-10052-4_3

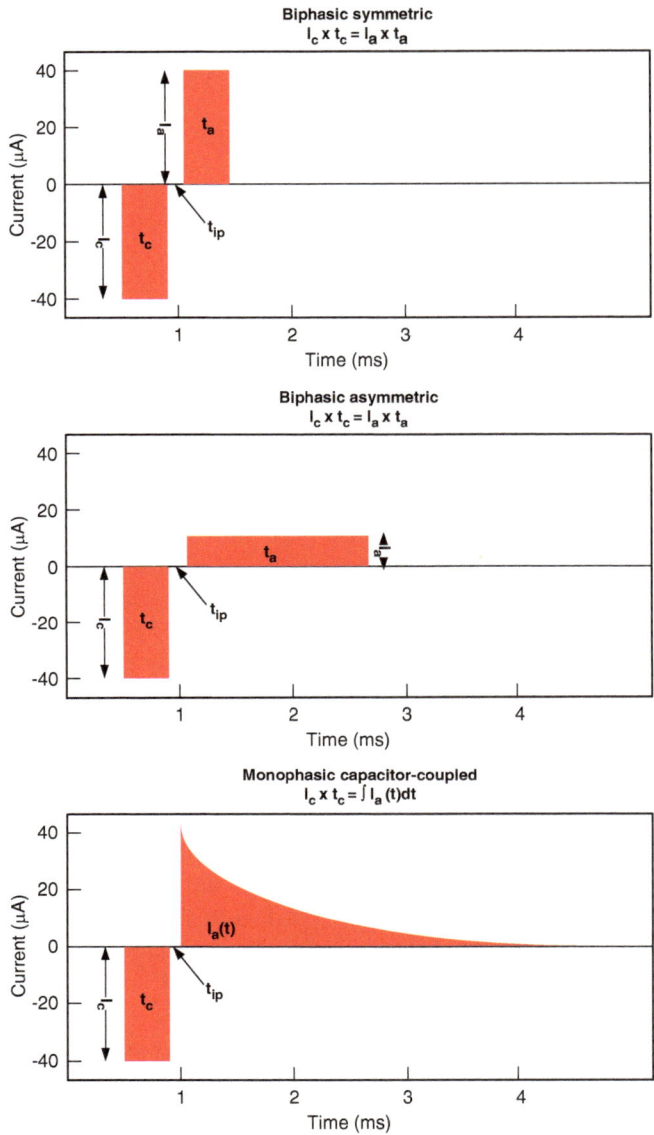

Fig. 3.1 Various biphasic charge balanced current pulses used in medical applications. I_c = cathodic current, I_a = anodic current, t_c = cathodic half-phase period, t_{ip} = interphase delay, t_a = anodic half-phase period. The idea for the figure is adapted from [1]

One major problem obeying the rule of symmetrical voltage on R_{FW} is that the forward and reverse reactions have different natures and different rates, i.e. R_{FW} value depends on the current polarity. The two reactions also don't occur at opposite phase boundary voltage drops, which is the result of the hysteresis

Fig. 3.2 The Randles
electrode model

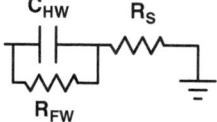

present in the electrode system due to the Nernst equation. Briefly said reversing the reaction does not require inverting the electrode potential but rather a reduction of the value is sufficient, as the products which are the reactants of the reverse reaction are already present at the electrode surface. A thorough discussion is out of the scope of this book.

Regarding above facts, determining a bi-phasic current pulse which fulfills the charge balance for the current into R_{FW} is impossible in practice.

For lower frequencies and slower signal waveforms, electrode model is more complicated than the Randles model. It has nonlinear characteristics which cannot be modeled by standard electrical elements having fixed values, like resistors and capacitors. Also incorporating non-linear elements like diodes may model some behaviors of the electrode-electrolyte interface like the dependence of the faradaic resistor on the interface voltage drop, but it cannot completely represent the reality.

Consider the cyclic voltammetry trace of electrically activated iridium oxide (the so called AIROF) which features reversible reactions (Fig. 3.3). The scan rate is very slow, so the dynamic behavior of the Helmholtz capacitance has a negligible effect on the measured trace. The positive peaks A and B correspond to two distinct oxidation reactions at the surface of the electrode, pertaining to different electrode potentials. The negative peaks C and D correspond to reduction reactions. C matches A and D matches B, as they have similar shape. The reduction potential peak (for example at C, E_{PC}) does not happen at a negative electrode-electrolyte voltage drop, but at a positive one even near to the potential where oxidation potential peak (at A, E_{PA}) is located. If the surface redox reactions are fast and the reaction rate is limited by the diffusion of the reactants in the solution, the difference between the oxidation and reduction peaks is only 59 mV/n for a reaction where n electrons are transferred in the stoichiometry of the reaction. This state is called electrochemical reversibility, which means that the thermodynamic equilibrium in the redox reaction at the surface is established fast at every applied electrode potential. Note that this concept is not the same as the chemical reversibility explained before. A system can be electrochemically irreversible but chemically reversible. As seen in Fig. 3.3, iridium oxide is already electrochemically irreversible even at the very slow potential ramp of 50 mV/s, as the $E_{PA} - E_{PC}$ is already larger than 59 mV.

In Fig. 3.3, after the voltage ramp is inverted, a negative current flows although a positive voltage is still existing between the working and the reference electrode (a three-electrode setup was used). This means that at this state, the electrode is supplying the rest of the system with power, i.e. it is working like a battery or voltage supply. Considering a slow biphasic anodic first current pulse injected into the electrode, if the first anodic pulse contains enough charge, it will change the electrode model to a model containing a voltage source in parallel to the interface capacitance. The limitation of the Randles model for this case is revealed.

Fig. 3.3 Cyclic voltammetry diagram for iridium oxide, the *blue area* is the so called cathodic charge storage capacity (CSC$_C$), original picture was taken from [1], with permission

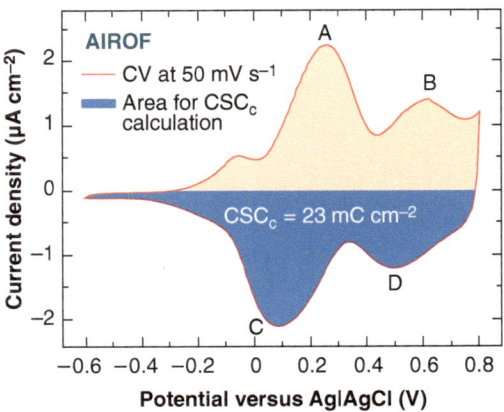

The total amount of charge available from the material at a given scan rate (working electrode voltage slope rate) is given by the area enclosed by the CV curve, the so called charge storage capacity (CSC). At very slow voltage ramps, iridium oxide injects most of the charge through redox reactions as can be seen in Fig. 3.3, so the C_{HW} in the Randles model can be neglected because of the relatively small parallel R_{FW}. The negative current explained above adds a hysteresis behavior to the model, i.e. the model contains an energy source depending on the charge injected into the electrode up to the current moment.

In many applications like in visual prostheses, charge injection into the electrodes result in much faster electrode-electrolyte interface voltage drop change rates than 50 mV/s. Measurements done here showed that injecting 18 nC charge into a disk iridium oxide electrode of 30 μm radius with a 1 ms long anodic +0.8 V amplitude pulse charges the interface capacitance to voltages in the orders of magnitude of hundreds of millivolts. This corresponds to a voltage ramp slope of hundreds of V/s for the cyclic voltammetry. As the redox reactions on iridium oxide are electrochemically irreversible, when the scan rate is increased, the anodic potential peak (E_{PA}) moves to right and the cathodic potential peak (E_{PC}) moves to the left. This occurs because the faradaic current needs more time to respond to the applied voltage. Figure 3.4 shows CV measurements with different scan rates in a 0.5 M H_2SO_4 solution. Note that the current magnitude here is normalized to the scan rate, i.e. for higher scan rates the actual current is larger than what it seems on the graph. The cathodic current peak actually vanishes at higher scan rates. For high scan rates, E_{PA} is proportional to the logarithm of the scan rate [6]. Consequently, at very high scan rates no peak is visible in the water window range (-0.6 V $\rightarrow$ $+0.8$ V). Furthermore, as the scan rate increases, the Helmholtz capacitor charging current of the electrode (sometimes called the background current) which is linearly proportional to the scan rate becomes the dominant contributor to the total electrode current. The cyclic voltammetry graph will then resemble that of a purely capacitive charge injection mechanism. For a large electrode with a surface of for example 1.4 cm^2, the charging and discharging

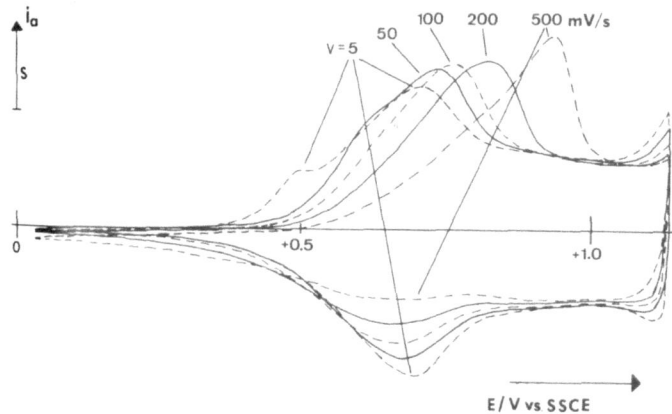

Fig. 3.4 Cyclic voltammetry diagram for iridium oxide for different scan rates, picture was taken from [6], with permission

at iridium surface is done mostly through the double layer capacitance and not through the electrochemical reactions already at a scan rate of only 200 mV/s [2]. In order to exploit the reversible chemical reactions, the electrode must be as small as possible.

At high scan rates, although the redox reactions have a lower effect on the available charge, due to the higher charging current the available CSC is increased. The water window itself does not depend considerably on the scan rate and thus on the signal frequency. Therefore, although more current can be injected, the voltage range (water window) remains the same.

Using slower signals (longer pulses) is generally not beneficial. In contrast to electrochemical reversibility, chemical reversibility requires fast signals, otherwise the reaction products diffuse away from the surface before being used in the reverse reaction.

The above discussion holds also for other materials like platinum, in which there are also current peaks corresponding to redox reactions at low scan rates. Again, with the typically short current pulses in neural stimulation, the redox reactions don't play a major role in charge injection, unless the electrode size is very small, i.e. has at least one dimension smaller than the surrounding diffusion layer. Therefore, in practice the simple model of Fig. 2.1b suffices. This means biphasic charge balanced current pulses (like the symmetrical ones) are actually the best option for electrode charge balance, especially for shorter stimulation pulses. The remaining residual voltage is removed after each pulse pair through methods explained in the following.

In order to maintain charge balance at electrode surface, in addition to using charge balanced, biphasic current pulses, the residual charge on the electrodes after the stimulation pulse must be eliminated. Charge-balancing methods are broken into three categories:

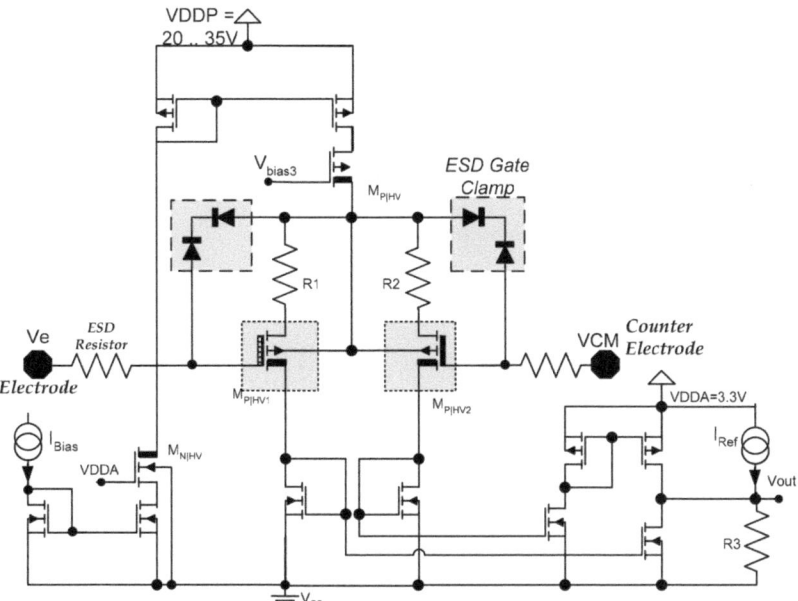

Fig. 3.5 Active charge balancer input stage from [5], picture used with permission ©2006 IEEE

- **Passive charge balancing**: Means connecting the electrodes to the counter electrode(s) after each biphasic pulse. This method has been used in [4, 7] to discharge the electrodes regularly and avoid build-up of high voltages on the electrodes. This method may not be effective to get rid of the excess charge if the discharge period is not long enough [8]. Therefore, other charge balancing methods are developed.

- **Using a current source for removing the residual charge**: In this method, a current source discharges the electrodes after stimulation towards the potential of the counter electrode. The current source is preferred to using a switch because the current is fixed and controlled so current spikes which would potentially cause undesired neural stimulation are avoided.

- **Active charge balancing**: An example was explained in [5]. The lack of high voltage ± 15 V transmission gates in the technology made using passive discharging impossible there. Therefore, an active discharging scheme was developed. Figure 3.5 shows the circuit used for the input stage of the active charge balancer. The residual charge remaining on the electrode after each anodic/cathodic pulse pair is dynamically measured with a differential voltage measurer. This value is processed and compared against an acceptable voltage window (± 50 mV in this case). If the value falls within this range, nothing extra occurs. If the value falls outside of the range, an acceptable charge packet is sent to the electrode to counter the charge before it becomes harmful to the surrounding tissue.

References

1. Cogan SF (2008) Neural stimulation and recording electrodes. Tech. rep., EIC Laboratories
2. Gilbert J, International A (2010) Medical Device Materials V: Proceedings of the Materials & Processes for Medical Devices Conference 2009, August 10–12, 2009, Minneapolis, MN, USA. Medical device materials, ASM International, URL http://books.google.de/books?id= LqQaGXFDdLsC
3. Krishnan A, Kelly S (2012) On the cause and control of residual voltage generated by electrical stimulation of neural tissue. In: Engineering in Medicine and Biology Society, EMBC, 2012 Annual International Conference of the IEEE
4. Lee C, Hsieh C (2011) A 0.8V 64x64 CMOS imager with integrated sense-and-stimulus pixel for artificial retina applications. In: Solid State Circuits Conference (A-SSCC), 2011 IEEE Asian, pp 193–196, DOI 10.1109/ASSCC.2011.6123635
5. Ortmanns M, Unger N, Rocke A, Gehrke M, Tietdke HJ (2006) A $0.1\,mm^2$, digitally programmable nerve stimulation pad cell with high-voltage capability for a retinal implant. In: IEEE International Solid-State Circuits Conference, pp 89–98
6. Pickup PG, Birss VI (1988) The kinetics of charging and discharging of iridium oxide films in aqueous and non-aqueous media. Journal of Electroanalytical Chemistry and Interfacial Electrochemistry 240(1–2):185–199, DOI http://dx.doi.org/10.1016/0022-0728(88)80322-X, URL http://www.sciencedirect.com/science/article/pii/002207288880322X
7. Rothermel A, Liu L, Aryan NP, Fischer M, Wünschmann J, Kibbel S, Harscher A (2009) A CMOS chip with active pixel array and specific test features for subretinal implantation. IEEE Journal of Solid-State Circuits 44(1):290–299
8. Sooksood K, Stieglitz T, Ortmanns M (2009) An experimental study on passive charge balancing. Advances in Radio Science 7:197–200, DOI 10.5194/ars-7-197-2009, URL http:// www.adv-radio-sci.net/7/197/2009/

Chapter 4
Primary Current Distribution and Electrode Geometry

The current density pattern on the surface of an electrode depends on the electrode shape and position [9, 11, 12, 14, 17]. It affects the corrosion behavior of the electrodes considerably. If electrode polarization is ignored, it was shown in [12] that on a disk electrode, with the surface in the same level as the surface of the surrounding insulator, the current density increases from the center of the disk while approaching the edge, with theoretically an infinite value at the edge. This assumption (no electrode polarization) can be made if the potential on the electrolyte side of the double layer is equal to that of the electrode. The current density under this condition is called **primary current distribution**. This state prevails at high frequency when the double layer capacitance behaves as a short circuit [14].

It has been demonstrated that the primary current distribution can have a considerable effect on electrochemical reactions at the electrode surface [14]. There are reports that patients undergoing electro-surgery sometimes suffer burns around the perimeter of the dispersive electrode, presumably because the primary current distribution achieves high current and charge densities at the electrode edge [14]. There is evidence that the edges of cochlear implant electrodes are sometimes the preferred site of corrosive attack [7, 15]. Nonuniform current density also raises the question of whether heating effects contribute to damage [14]. Ordinary patch electrodes used for internal cardiac defibrillation conduct a substantial portion of the current along electrode periphery which can result in burns because of the ohmic heating of the tissue [2].

Primary current distribution exists especially when a current or a voltage step is applied [1, 3, 14, 16]. Therefore, ramp current waveforms with lower slopes or sine wave stimulus are superior compared to square pulses regarding corrosion and uniform cell stimulation [1]. In the following, first the effect of different geometrical modifications of electrodes on the current distribution is theoretically investigated. Then, a short list of changes which would potentially improve the corrosion behavior of electrodes is suggested.

© The Author(s) 2015
N. Pour Aryan et al., *Stimulation and Recording Electrodes for Neural Prostheses*,
SpringerBriefs in Electrical and Computer Engineering 78,
DOI 10.1007/978-3-319-10052-4_4

4.1 The Effect of Electrode Recession on Current Distribution

Recessed electrodes have a more uniform current distribution both at the electrode-electrolyte interface and at the carrier-tissue junction [9, 11, 14]. For patient's safety, clinical use of recessed electrodes in cochlear implants is recommended [14].

A disk electrode recessed by an amount equal to its radius has an approximately uniform current distribution on it (with 2 % variation from the average) [11, 14]. A recession amount of 0.3 times the radius causes already a much more uniform current distribution compared to a surface mounted electrode with no recession [14]. A detailed solution of Laplace's equation corresponding to the system of a recessed disk electrode in a semi-infinite space of finite resistivity ρ was done in [14] (Fig. 4.1). Here "I" is the injected current. Figure 4.2 illustrates the results. In this figure the normalized current densities are plotted versus the distance from electrode center for different recession depths. This shows a dramatic improvement in the current distribution with even slight recession depths. These small depths would pose little additional difficulty to the fabrication of electrodes given this substantial reduction in current density at the edge [14]. The current delivered to neurons remains constant as the total injected current remains the same as with an unrecessed electrode [14]. According to [11], with a recession depth of only 0.1 times the radius of disk electrode, the peak current density reduces to at most 43 % of the peak current of a surface mounted disk electrode with the same radius and total injected current. For $0.4 \times Disk\ radius$ recession, this peak current reduces to just 30 % of that of an unrecessed electrode.

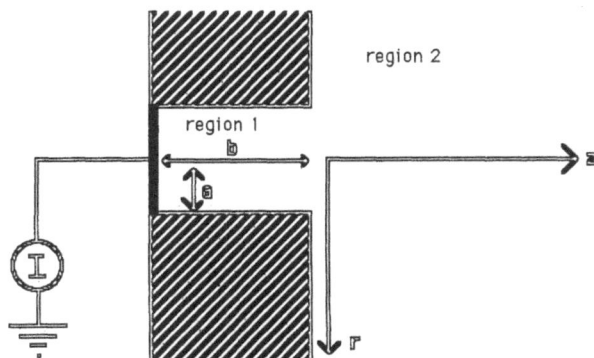

Fig. 4.1 System of the recessed disk electrode investigated in [14], the right half-space has resistivity ρ. Picture from [14], with permission ©1987 IEEE

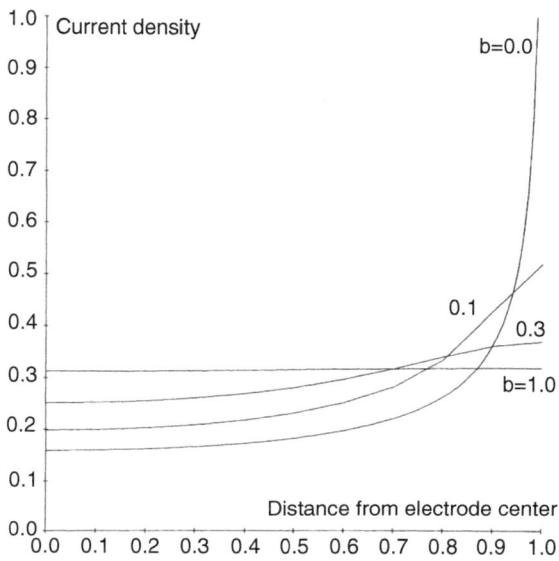

Fig. 4.2 Current density on the surface of the disk for various recession depths, b = recession depth, electrode radius = 1, injected total current I =1 A. Medium's resistivity is arbitrary. Data from [14], with permission ©1987 IEEE

4.2   Geometric Shape and the Current Distribution

The geometric shape of the electrode influences the current distribution too. Only a hemispherical metal electrode on the surface of a flat insulator of infinite extent (Fig. 4.3) has exactly uniform primary current distribution across the surface [11]. This was the type of electrode used by Brummer and Turner to estimate the maximum surface redox limits for platinum, considering the size of their electrode carrier [4–6]. Nonspherical electrodes may be operating irreversibly even when established "safe" stimulation parameters are used [14]. With the addition of microstructures (micro-post structures) on the electrode surface, current crowding tends to occur near the sharp convex corners. The increased current density at these sites leads to higher irrecoverable charge loss and more corrosion [10].

A rectangular shape is typically not an appropriate geometry for a flat electrode from current distribution point of view [13, 14]. In an array of rectangular electrodes with the counter electrode nearby, Iain Henly et al. [8] showed that the current density on the corners of a rectangular electrode can be considerably higher than other points on the sides of the rectangle away from the corners. This is because voltage drop on the electrode-electrolyte interface is higher on the edges and even higher at the corners and lower in the middle when the electrode potential changes abruptly.

A uniform current density electrode was designed in [11] by combining the shapes of a hemispherical electrode and a recessed electrode. This electrode had

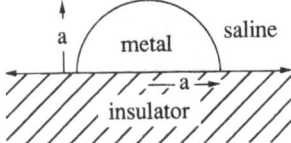

Fig. 4.3 A hemispherical electrode, picture from [11], with permission ©1992 IEEE

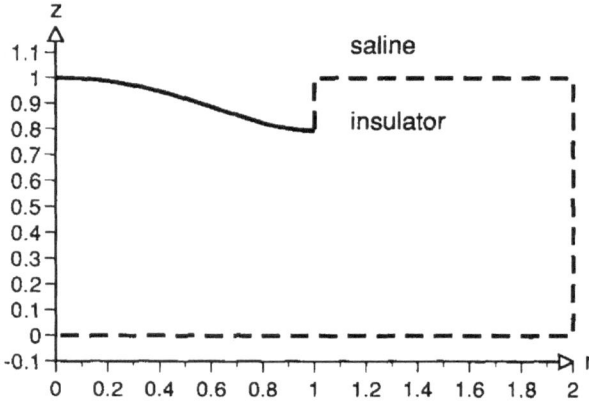

Fig. 4.4 Radial section of a uniform current minimum profile electrode. The metal is shown with a *solid line* and the saline-insulator interface is shown with a *dashed line*. From [11], with permission ©1992 IEEE

some curvature and was mounted at the bottom of a shallow cylindrical insulating well. The electrode height was equal to the recession depth. The radial section of the electrode on an insulator carrier having a radius two times that of the electrode is depicted in Fig. 4.4.

As a summary, the following modifications can be applied to electrodes to enforce a more uniform surface current density and therefore less corrosion susceptibility and higher patient safety:

- Recessing the electrodes into insulating wells. In the case of disk electrodes a recession of 0.1–0.4 times the disk radius has already major positive effects, the more the recession depth the better. The required depth in the case of rectangular electrodes is not mentioned in the literature, but the positive influence of recession on current distribution is certain.
- Disk shape is preferred to square.
- Adding some smooth curvature to the electrodes, like the electrodes designed in [11] (Fig. 4.4). Sharp convex corners must be avoided.

The most safe and at the same time conservative way to prevent harmful reactions at the electrode surface caused by non-uniform current distribution is to limit the electrode potential (in a two-electrode system the counter electrode is the potential reference) inside the water window, instead of limiting the interface capacitance voltage drop. It means the access voltage effect is neglected. In the current study, a hardware fulfilling this criterion was built and used to evaluate charge injection capacity for different materials. This is explained in the next chapter.

References

1. Ahuja AK, Behrend MR, Whalen JJ, Humayun MS, Weiland JD (2008) The dependence of spectral impedance on disc microelectrode radius. Biomedical Engineering, IEEE Transactions on 55(4):1457–1460, DOI 10.1109/TBME.2007.912430
2. Barnett DW, Fahy JB, Wu HJ, Lytle A, Kim Y (1988) Finite element model applications in defibrillation and external cardiac pacing. In: Engineering in Medicine and Biology Society, 1988. Proceedings of the Annual International Conference of the IEEE, pp 200–201 vol. 1, DOI 10.1109/IEMBS.1988.94477
3. Behrend MR, Ahuja AK, Weiland JD (2008) Dynamic current density of the disk electrode double-layer. Biomedical Engineering, IEEE Transactions on 55(3):1056–1062, DOI 10.1109/TBME.2008.915723
4. Brummer S, Turner M (1975) Electrical stimulation of the nervous system: The principle of safe charge injection with noble metal electrodes. Bioelectrochemistry and Bioenergetics 2(1):13–25, DOI 10.1016/0302-4598(75)80002-X, URL http://www.sciencedirect.com/science/article/pii/030245987580002X
5. Brummer SB, Turner MJ (1977a) Electrical stimulation with Pt electrodes: A method for determination of "real" electrode areas. Biomedical Engineering, IEEE Transactions on BME-24(5):436–439, DOI 10.1109/TBME.1977.326178
6. Brummer SB, Turner MJ (1977b) Electrochemical considerations for safe electrical stimulation of the nervous system with platinum electrodes. Biomedical Engineering, IEEE Transactions on BME-24(1):59–63, DOI 10.1109/TBME.1977.326218
7. Clark GM, Shepherd RK, Patrick JF, Black RC, Tong YC (1983) Design and fabrication of the banded electrode arraya. Annals of the New York Academy of Sciences 405(1):191–201, DOI 10.1111/j.1749-6632.1983.tb31632.x, URL http://dx.doi.org/10.1111/j.1749-6632.1983.tb31632.x
8. Henley IE, Fisher AC (2003) Computational electrochemistry: The simulation of voltammetry in microchannels with low conductivity solutions. The Journal of Physical Chemistry B 107(27):6579–6585, DOI 10.1021/jp030238k, URL http://pubs.acs.org/doi/abs/10.1021/jp030238k, http://pubs.acs.org/doi/pdf/10.1021/jp030238k
9. Humayun MS (2001) Intraocular retinal prosthesis
10. Hung A, Zhou D, Greenberg R, Judy J (2003) Dynamic electrochemical simulation of micromachined electrodes for neural-stimulation systems. In: Neural Engineering, 2003. Conference Proceedings. First International IEEE EMBS Conference on, pp 200–203, DOI 10.1109/CNE.2003.1196792
11. Ksienski DA (1992) A minimum profile uniform current density electrode. Biomedical Engineering, IEEE Transactions on 39(7):682–692, DOI 10.1109/10.142643
12. Newman J (1966) Resistance for flow of current to a disk. Journal of the electrochemical society, May, 501–502
13. Rubinstein JT (1988) Quasi-static analytical models of electrodes and electrode arrays for electrical stimulation of the cochlea, auditory nerve and cochlear nucleus. Thesis, University of Washington
14. Rubinstein JT, Spelman FA, Soma M, Suesserman MF (1987) Current density profiles of surface mounted and recessed electrodes for neural prostheses. Biomedical Engineering, IEEE Transactions on BME-34(11):864–875, DOI 10.1109/TBME.1987.326007

15. Shepherd RK, Murray MT, Hougiton ME, Clark GM (1985) Scanning electron microscopy of chronically stimulated platinum intracochlear electrodes. Biomaterials 6(4):237–242, DOI 10.1016/0142-9612(85)90019-5, URL http://www.sciencedirect.com/science/article/pii/0142961285900195
16. Wang B, Weiland JD (2012) Reduction of current density at disk electrode periphery by shaping current pulse edges. In: Engineering in Medicine and Biology Society (EMBC), 2012 Annual International Conference of the IEEE, pp 5138–5141, DOI 10.1109/EMBC.2012.6347150
17. Wiley JD, Webster JG (1982) Analysis and control of the current distribution under circular dispersive electrodes. Biomedical Engineering, IEEE Transactions on BME-29(5):381–385, DOI 10.1109/TBME.1982.324910

Chapter 5
Experiments Hardware and Methods

Three materials were extensively experimented with throughout the research here: TiN, iridium and iridium oxide (IrOx). The solution used in the experiments to mimic the surrounding tissue in the application is phosphate buffered saline (PBS). Before continuing with the investigation of different electrode materials and their characteristics, the hardware and methods developed and used here are explained briefly.

5.1 Fabrication and Processing of Micro Electrode Arrays (MEAs)

The MEAs are manufactured using thin film lithography on a float glass substrate. Gold lines are patterned with a lift-off technique on the surface of the substrate. The metal lines are covered with a polyimide insulation layer. A hard mask is used to remove the polyimide at the electrode sites and over the conduction pads. The TiN or iridium electrodes are patterned in a subsequent lift-off process. The profile of one electrode is shown in Fig. 5.1. The polyimide (PI) coating used for protection is resistant to most acids and alcohols, but it is not resistant to hydrolysis. A photograph of an electrode field of an iridium MEA containing 64 square electrodes is shown in Fig. 5.2. In this type of MEA, every four electrodes are connected via a gold line to a connection pad. Every electrode has an area of $50 \times 50 \, \mu m$. Figure 5.3 shows a MEA piece.

Another group of iridium MEAs which were used for extensive modeling and activation investigations were two standard Multi Channel Systems MEAs with round electrodes having a diameter of $30 \, \mu m$ (Fig. 8.2). These electrodes were accessible individually. In addition to the disc shaped microelectrodes, there was per MEA one large trapezoidal macroelectrode with an area of around $7 \, mm^2$, which

© The Author(s) 2015
N. Pour Aryan et al., *Stimulation and Recording Electrodes for Neural Prostheses*,
SpringerBriefs in Electrical and Computer Engineering 78,
DOI 10.1007/978-3-319-10052-4_5

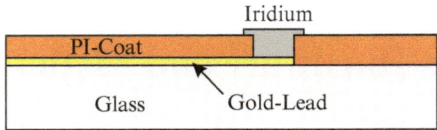

Fig. 5.1 Profile of MEA [4] ©2012 IEEE

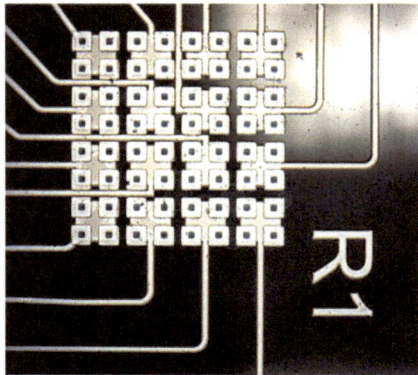

Fig. 5.2 Part of a MEA containing 64 electrodes. Every four electrodes are connected together and through a gold lead wire to a connection pad (see below)

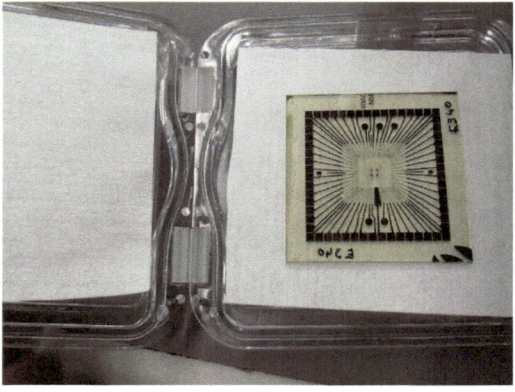

Fig. 5.3 A TiN MEA including 4 × 64 electrodes (the four small squares in the *middle*) and 60 pads on the sides

would usually be used as a counter electrode. In this study the macroelectrode was also used as an electrode under investigation to analyze the behavior of a large iridium electrode.

A two part silver conductive adhesive (EPOTEK H20E) and a paint brush (Fig. 5.4) were used for connecting the pads via enameled wires to connection sockets. The wire pieces are stripped at both ends and are fixed by sticky tapes on a connection setup.

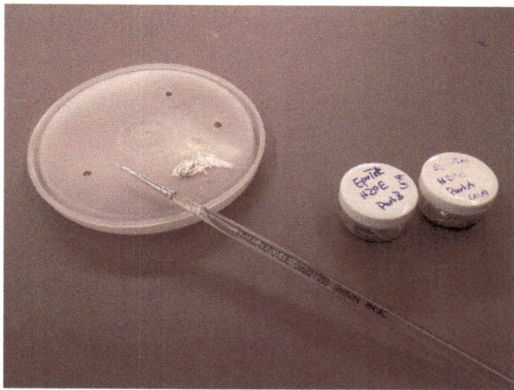

Fig. 5.4 Wiring connection tools

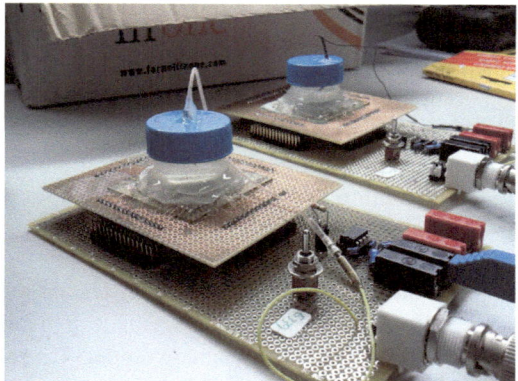

Fig. 5.5 Two vessels containing the corresponding MEAs and PBS plugged on two electrode accessing circuits

After the connection to the socket strips is done, a vessel formed by a plastic cylinder is used to enclose the electrodes. A glass ring and silicone (MED 1100 from Nusil, although other cheaper silicones like the UHU or Sylgard may also be applied) are used to seal the resulting vessel which is then filled with PBS. A plastic cap having a helical thread was perforated and a counter electrode was inserted and fixed into the resulting hole by silicone. The counter electrode had a relatively large area of $0.5\,\text{cm}^2$. To avoid any galvanic effects in lifetime experiments, the counter electrode was always chosen the same material as the electrodes under investigation, i.e. TiN for TiN microelectrodes and iridium for iridium or iridium oxide microelectrodes. A simple circuit is built on breadboard to connect a BNC plug to the electrodes under the test. Accessing the electrodes is done by jumpers. This setup is shown in Fig. 5.5.

5.2   The Developed Arbitrary Generator (AWG) Circuit

In the experiments, biphasic first-cathodic current pulses with arbitrary length and amplitudes were injected into each electrode. The electrodes were discharged after the end of the anodic pulse to remove the residual charge. To prevent large current spikes due to connecting the electrodes directly to the ground, a 1 kΩ resistor was used in series with the low resistance switch. The switch used is MAX319 (from Maxim Integrated Products Inc.) which is controlled by a TTL signal.

The hardware comprises a laptop, NI-6259 National Instruments multifunctional board, SCC-68 connection block and additional hardware to inject controlled current signals and limit the output voltage. A LabVIEW program generates biphasic voltage pulses through the NI-6259 board which are output to SCC-68 pins. It also generates the TTL signals which drive the switches (Fig. 5.6).

The system block-diagram is seen in Fig. 5.7. The voltage generated by the LabVIEW software and the NI system is converted to current by a voltage-current converter to generate current pulses with adjustable amplitudes and lengths. The rise and fall times of the pulse edges is also adjustable by the software. The stimulator circuit is designed to accommodate various voltage boundaries at the output, which was implemented by a voltage limiter. As lower electrode potential swings presumably result in longer electrode lifetime and lower stimulation power loss, this feature makes finding the minimum voltage swing required for a predefined charge injection value possible.

The system hardware is illustrated in Fig. 5.8.

The voltage-current converter is shown in Fig. 5.9. The op-amps used here were AD713 from Analog Devices. The input buffer was used to avoid the V-I converter from loading the SCC-68 connection block analog output. The relationship between the output current and the input voltage is:

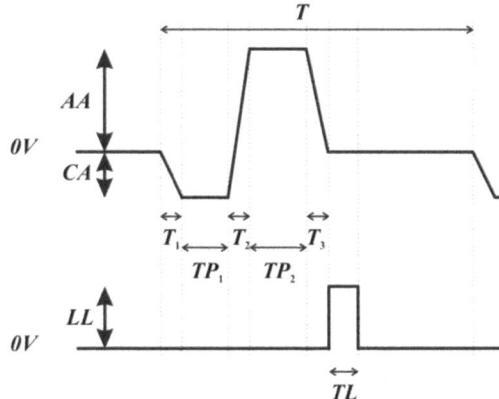

Fig. 5.6 Quasi-arbitrary voltage waveform generated inside LabVIEW and used for the AWG hardware of the system (*top*); digital signal used to turn the discharge switch on (*bottom*) [5] ©2012 IEEE

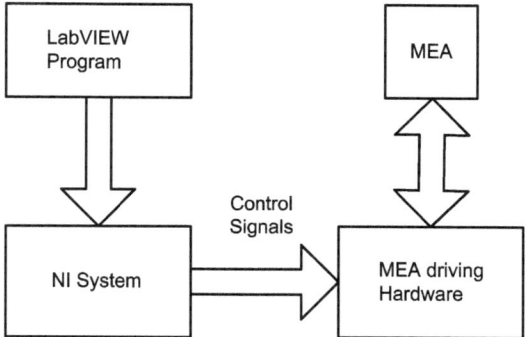

Fig. 5.7 The block-diagram of the system built to generate and measure current pulses and limit output voltage [5] ©2012 IEEE

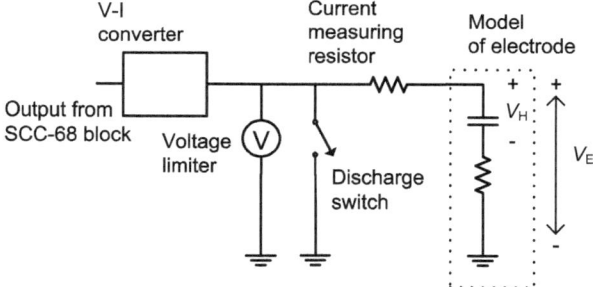

Fig. 5.8 The additional hardware built to generate and measure current and limit output voltage, picture adapted from [5] ©2012 IEEE

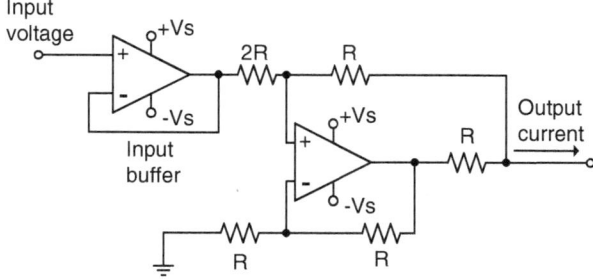

Fig. 5.9 The V-I converter [5]

To output
load

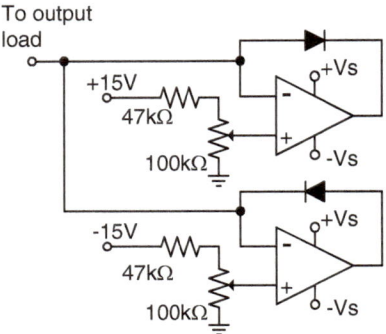

Fig. 5.10 Voltage limiter circuit [5]

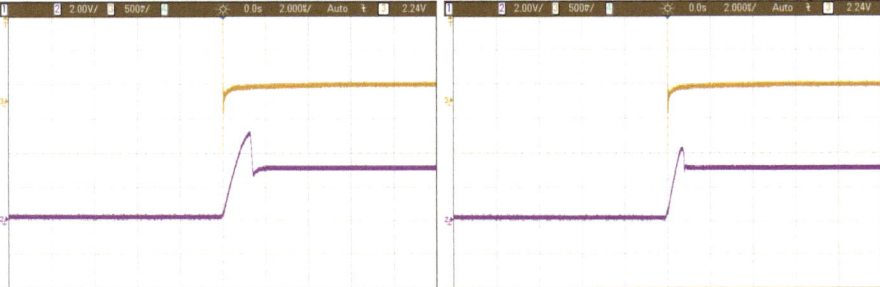

Fig. 5.11 Output voltage overshoot exceeding the positive voltage boundary is smaller with a
faster op-amp in the voltage clamp circuit. *Top picture* corresponds to AD713 (slew rate under
unity gain: $20\,V/\mu s$). *Bottom picture* corresponds to TLE2074CN (slew rate: $38\,V/\mu s$). Channel
2 (violet) is the output voltage. The input voltage from SCC-68 connection block is (0 and 1 V).
Channel 3 (*orange*) is the discharge signal and is not relevant here. The load is $10\,k\Omega$ resistor and
$100\,nF$ capacitor in series

$$I_{out} = \frac{V_{in}}{R}$$

In order to reduce losses and to maximize the number of units supportable by a
commercial DC power supply, the op-amp output current was minimized by setting
R to $1\,k\Omega$.

The voltage limiter circuit is shown in Fig. 5.10. This circuit limits the output
(electrode) voltage inside the boundaries set by the two trimmer potentiometers.
The negative and positive boundaries are adjustable to values in the ranges of
$-10\,V \rightarrow 0\,V$ and $0\,V \rightarrow 10\,V$, respectively.

If a high enough input voltage step is applied from the input SCC-68 pin, the
output voltage may exceed the voltage limit for a short time because the op-amp is
not fast enough to turn the corresponding diode immediately on. A faster op-amp
like TLE2074CN (with higher slew rate) makes this overshoot (or undershoot)
smaller (Fig. 5.11).

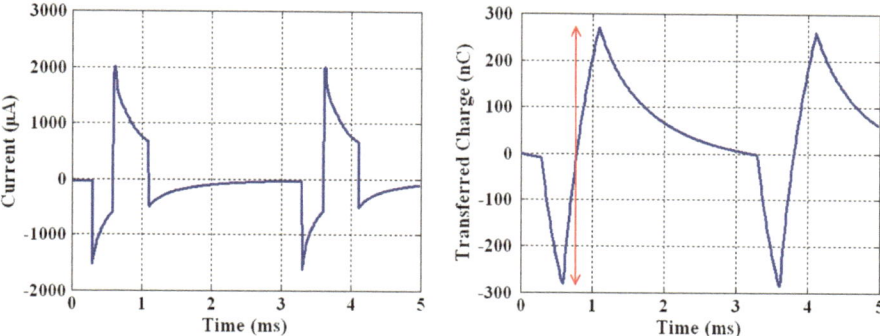

Fig. 5.12 Transferred charge (*right*) was calculated by LabVIEW by integrating the current (*left*) resulting from a biphasic rectangular ±2 V voltage on the electrodes. Charge injection capacity here corresponds to the anodic phase current. Sixteen 50 × 50 μm iridium electrodes were connected here. The total anodic charge injection marked by the *red arrow* is about 560 nC

5.3   Charge Injection Capacity Measurement

As mentioned above charge injection capacity is the amount of charge injected into the solution per pulse in a given water window. Charge injection capacity depends on the signal timing. As in our application (subretinal stimulator) periodic biphasic current or voltage waveforms with a cathodic pulse length of 0.3 ms and anodic pulse length of 0.5 ms are typical, they were used to extract the charge injection capacity in every case. The resulting current was measured by a resistor in series with the electrode under test. Electrode voltage boundaries were set by the voltage limiter.

In order to have a consistent method in all experiments, the integral of the current injected in the anodic phase was always considered as charge injection capacity. Figure 5.12 shows the concept.

5.4   Impedance Spectroscopy

In impedance spectroscopy electrode impedance composed of amplitude and phase is measured by putting a sine voltage with varying frequency on the electrode and measuring the resulting current amplitude and phase shift over the frequency. Electrode model can be extracted from the resulting impedance data. A professional potentiostat was used for impedance spectroscopy and cyclic voltammetry. Electrodes were tested in a two electrode cell arrangement, i.e. working (electrode under investigation) and counter electrodes. The counter electrode had a very large area compared to the microelectrodes under test (0.5 cm^2 compared to 706.5 μm^2, disk electrodes used), as it is the situation in the monopolar stimulation structure used very often in practice. Therefore, the counter electrode impedance could be neglected as its interface capacitance was very large and it had little contribution to the series spreading resistance because of its large area. Moreover, for impedance spectroscopy the sine voltage has a very low amplitude as will be explained in the following, thus the current flowing from the working to the counter electrode is small. Consequently, the voltage drop on the counter electrode impedance is negligible and does not affect the measurement considerably. Therefore, a two electrode system arrangement provides a sufficient accuracy in this case. In this arrangement, the working and working sense terminals of the potentiostat are connected together. The reference and counter electrode terminals are connected to form the pseudo-reference electrode of the two electrode cell.

If the electrode under test be large as for example the macroelectrode used in deep brain stimulation applications, a three electrode cell arrangement must be used in order to eliminate the effect of counter electrode impedance on the measurement. A reference electrode, usually a silver-silver chloride electrode, must be purchased and connected to the potentiostat. The three electrode setup was explained in Chap. 1.

In the potentiostat's software setup, the reference for impedance spectroscopy was always set to the open circuit potential (OCP). This is the voltage that exists between the working and counter electrodes when no net current flows, no load is connected and the system is in thermodynamic equilibrium. Thermodynamic equilibrium was always established after a relatively short time of around 20 s. Random OCP values were measured by the potentiostat during the tests, lying in the range from $-400\,mV \rightarrow 350\,mV$. This means that here the OCP potential was not set by the electrochemical cell but rather by the measurement setup. As it is seen the average OCP lied near zero. This was expected as the counter electrode was always chosen to be from the same material as the microelectrodes under test, i.e. an iridium counter electrode for iridium or iridium oxide microelectrodes. Actually in this case one could also choose the counter electrode as the reference. However, if different materials be chosen, a non-zero average OCP potential builds up due to the galvanic effects.

If OCP is to be considered as the reference when the working and the counter electrodes are from the same material and from the same batch of fabrication process, the two can be connected together for some time until they reach a stable equilibrium with the electrolyte, i.e. OCP approaches zero.

The measured impedance amplitude and phase can be used to approximate the electrode model. This can be either done by using curve fitting softwares or by applying analytical methods. Consider for example the previously mentioned Randles model of Fig. 3.2. The total impedance (Z) of this model is equal to:

$$Z = R_S + \left(R_{FW} \| \frac{1}{jC_{HW}\omega} \right) = R_S + \frac{R_{FW}}{1 + jR_{FW}C_{HW}\omega} \tag{5.1}$$

Here, $\omega = 2\pi f$ is the angular frequency and j is the imaginary unit.

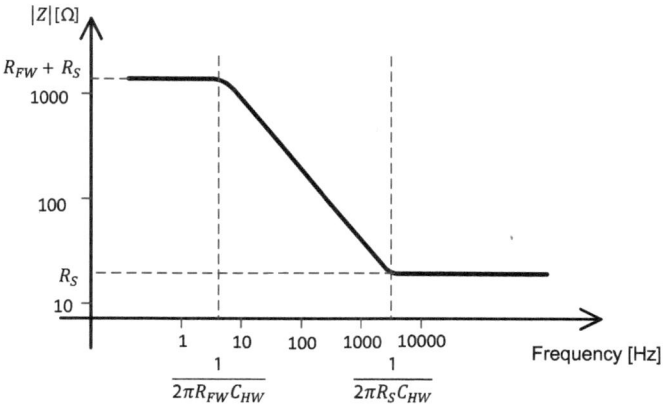

Fig. 5.13 Impedance amplitude versus frequency for an electrode having a Randles model

If the electrode size and material let the frequency range to cover the whole electrode details in the impedance spectrum, the measured impedance amplitude versus frequency would look like seen in Fig. 5.13. The values for R_S, R_{FW} and C_{HW} can be read off and calculated from the saturation values and corner frequencies as marked in the figure.

5.4.1 Linear Range for Excitation Voltage Amplitude

For impedance spectroscopy, the dependence of the measured current on the applied voltage must be linear. Usually in the literature a low enough amplitude between 10 and 100 mV is chosen for the exciting voltage [1, 3, 7]. It is assumed that the operation is in a linear region. To determine the linear range in the current application to exclude any error possibility, impedance spectroscopy was performed for a single electrode and the impedance amplitude versus frequency was plotted for different excitation sine wave amplitudes as illustrated in Fig. 5.14. As can be seen in the figure, below 200 mV the impedance amplitude curves are similar. Above 200 mV signal amplitude, the spectra start to deviate from the ones under this limit. So the excitation voltage to measured current relationship begins to become nonlinear at 200 mV. Impedance spectroscopy was done several times with the same electrode using the signal amplitude of 10 mV and a maximum average standard deviation of 1 % was observed in the measurements. This means the signal to noise ratio is high enough for 10 mV signal amplitude. Therefore, a voltage amplitude of 10 mV is used for impedance spectroscopy measurements in the following.

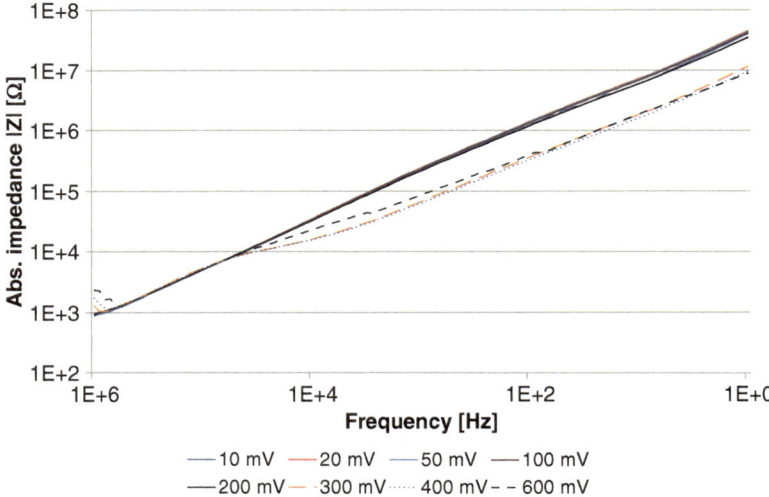

Fig. 5.14 Under an excitation sine voltage amplitude of 200 mV, the absolute impedance versus frequency is relatively independent from the excitation voltage amplitude. Thus, under this boundary, the excitation voltage to measured current relationship is linear. The frequency axis is labeled as in the measurements, from higher down to the lower frequencies

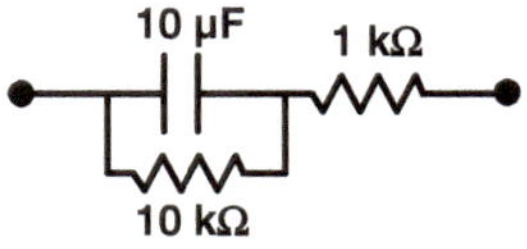

Fig. 5.15 Circuit corresponding to the test cell accompanying the potentiostat

The above method can be used to determine the linear range for signal voltage amplitude in recording electrodes.

5.4.2 Potentiostat Limits and the Measurement Frequency Range

Although in literature a frequency range from 1 Hz to 1 MHz is common for impedance spectroscopy [1, 3, 7], preliminary electrode measurements showed unexpected results which could not be explained by any acceptable electrode model. An experiment was done using the test cell (dummy cell) accompanying the potentiostat to verify its functionality. Figure 5.15 shows the corresponding circuit.

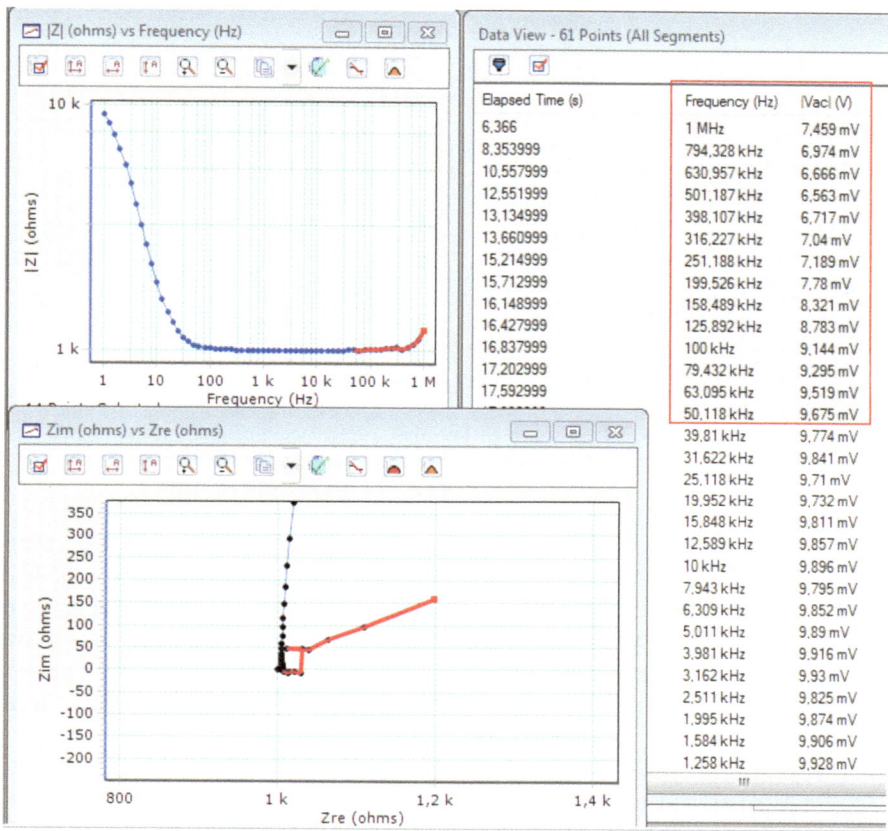

Fig. 5.16 Screenshot of the AC dummy cell impedance spectroscopy measurement results for the frequency range from 1 Hz to 1 MHz

Figure 5.16 shows a screen shot of the impedance spectroscopy measurement result. Here a sine voltage amplitude of 10 mV was used. Above right it can be seen that the potentiostat is not able to exert a constant sine wave amplitude to the electrode for higher frequencies. Above left an increase in the impedance amplitude for higher frequencies is observed (inductive behavior, section marked by red color), which is not possible for a cell consisting only of resistor and capacitor. The red marked portion of the plotted Nyquist plot (bottom left) belongs to high frequencies. This is also unexpected because in this range the capacitor of the dummy cell is almost shorted, so the impedance should not have an imaginary part.

It was shown in [6] that inductive impedance measured at high frequencies (above 10 kHz) in impedance spectroscopy is largely due to the input capacitance of the reference electrode connection of the potentiostat. This capacitance is typically around 5 pF. This artifact is general to all the potentiostats. This behavior is particularly enhanced when the electrode under test has high capacitance, as

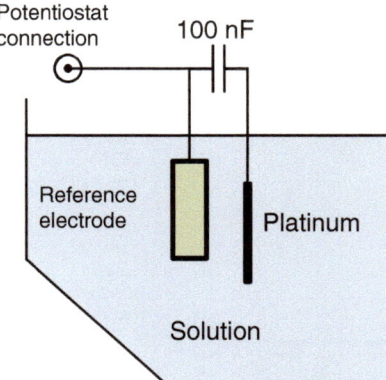

Fig. 5.17 Eliminating the effect of a high impedance reference electrode on impedance spectroscopy by compensating the low pass characteristic through an additional capacitor

in iridium oxide electrodes, or when the reference electrode has a high series resistance, for example when Luggin capillaries are used. In these cases, the high series resistance of the reference electrode combined with the input capacitance of the reference electrode terminal of the potentiostat cause the artifact. It was shown in [2] that using an extra path for the AC signal through an additional platinum electrode coupled to the main reference electrode by a 100 nF capacitor eliminates this problem (see Fig. 5.17).

As a summary, the measurement setup used in the current study was inaccurate for frequencies above 50 kHz. Therefore, the upper limit for the measurements in the following chapters was set to 50 kHz. On the other hand, investigations showed that frequencies lower than 1 Hz (down to 0.001 Hz) do not provide new information about the electrodes behavior here while they make the experiment duration considerably longer. So the frequency range was limited to between 1 Hz and 50 kHz.

References

1. Cogan SF (2008) Neural stimulation and recording electrodes. Tech. rep., EIC Laboratories
2. Mansfeld F, Lin S, Chen Y, Shih H (1988) Minimization of high-frequency phase shifts in impedance measurements. Tech. rep.
3. Poppendieck W (2010) Untersuchungen zum Einsatz neuer Elektrodenmaterialien: Und deren Evaluation als Reiz- und Ableitelektrode. Südwestdeutscher Verlag, URL http://books.google.de/books?id=Z1xnRwAACAAJ
4. Pour Aryan N, Brendler C, Rieger V, Schleehauf S, Heusel G, Rothermel A (2012a) In vitro study of iridium electrodes for neural stimulation. In: Engineering in Medicine and Biology Society,EMBC, 2012 Annual International Conference of the IEEE

5. Pour Aryan N, Rieger V, Brendler C, Rothermel A (2012b) An economical and convenient experiment setup for electrode investigation. In: Engineering in Medicine and Biology Society,EMBC, 2012 Annual International Conference of the IEEE
6. Vanysek P, Birss V (2000) Potentiostat-induced artifacts in impedance measurements. Tech. rep., Northern Illinois University
7. Weiland JD, Anderson DJ (2000) Chronic neural stimulation with thin-film, iridium oxide electrodes. Biomedical Engineering, IEEE Transactions on 47(7):911–918, DOI 10.1109/10. 846685

Chapter 6
Electrode Materials: State-of-the-Art and Experiments

Platinum is the most commonly used electrode material. The charge injection limit for platinum electrodes was found to be $400\,\mu C/cm^2$ in [4]. Tim Boretius et al. have reported a value of only $75\,\mu C/cm^2$ [3]. Platinum electrodes have proven success in practice, for example in many cochlear implants. Because of their relatively low charge injection capacity, they are usually used where large electrodes are applicable as in intracortical implant [8]. The limit for neural stimulation regarding tissue safety has been determined to be $1\,mC/cm^2$. In order to increase the charge injection capacity of platinum, various approaches have been proposed in the past few decades, like the galvanization of platinum black or gray. Although platinum black possesses a highly porous layer and therefore high charge injection capacity, its deposition often requires a lead containing electrolyte which limits its application because of cytotoxicity concerns. Other ways to increase the active area include electrochemical deposition of third-party components like oxides and nitrides (IrOx, Ta_2O_5, TiN) or conducting polymer coatings (PEDOT) [3]. Although this may increase the charge injection capacity, a higher composition of materials is resulted, which may lead to galvanic effects and subsequently corrosion and delamination. No connections within an implant system that are exposed to tissue is allowed to be of dissimilar metals. The only exception is Pt to Pt/Ir system [29].

In systems involving activated iridium (iridium oxide) electrodes and gold conductor lines underneath, sputtered platinum can be used as an intermediate layer to protect the gold from corroding and dissolving into the solution. Iridium oxide is a highly porous material, providing micro-pores through which gold would otherwise interact with the solution. In [34] a 150 nm thick intermediate platinum layer separates a 500 nm thick iridium oxide electrode material from the $3\,\mu m$ thick underlying gold wiring.

To avoid any risk of galvanic corrosion, Tim Boretius et al. have introduced a new method of generating porous platinum surfaces by electrochemically depositing a platinum-copper alloy and a subsequent dissolution of copper [3] using cyclic

© The Author(s) 2015
N. Pour Aryan et al., *Stimulation and Recording Electrodes for Neural Prostheses*, SpringerBriefs in Electrical and Computer Engineering 78,
DOI 10.1007/978-3-319-10052-4_6

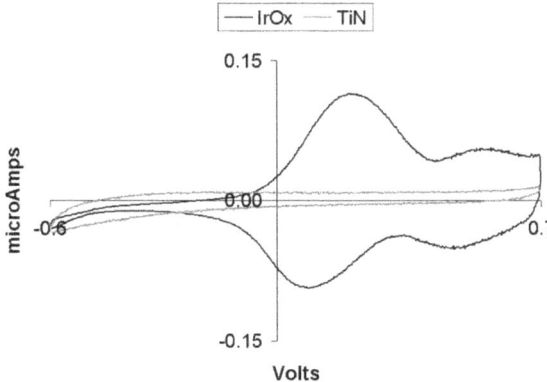

Fig. 6.1 Cyclic voltammogram for IrOx and TiN (from [32], with permission ©2002 IEEE), the reference electrode was a saturated calomel electrode

voltammetry. The electrodes exhibited an increased porosity of about 238 times more than sputtered platinum. The electrode impedance characteristics was reported to resemble those of platinum black and iridium oxide.

In recent years, both iridium oxide and titanium nitride have undergone much experimentation to determine if they could safely deliver more charge per unit area than platinum electrodes. TiN is already commonly used in integrated circuit fabrication, so using it as an electrode material does not require any new deposition methods to be developed [32]. A cyclic voltammogram of both materials (Fig. 6.1) uncovers the nature of the charge transfer in the electrode. The peaks in the IrOx graph show that IrOx delivers most of its charge from redox reactions involving the oxidation and reduction of the iridium oxide itself. The area encircled by the cyclic voltammogram is a measure of the maximum charge available from the material, although due to chemical reactions rate limits and pore resistance only some fraction of it is available for electrostimulation. The graph shows that IrOx can store more charge than TiN. IrOx can deliver more charge per unit area than TiN except in high frequencies. The redox reactions on IrOx surface were found to be completely reversible. The smooth rectangular TiN curve reveals that the current from the electrode is primarily non-faradaic (capacitive) [32].

The limits of safe charge injection regarding electrode integrity were determined based on the assumed water window. When the electrode potential is within this range, hydrolysis, which is potentially dangerous, theoretically does not occur. In [32], the safe limit was found to be $4\,mC/cm^2$ for IrOx. TiN was shown to be able to deliver $950\,\mu C/cm^2$ with anodic current and $550\,\mu C/cm^2$ with cathodic current pulses. All of these values were found using a $0.2\,ms$ current pulse and $4,000\,\mu m^2$ electrodes [32]. Therefore, both TiN and IrOx have higher charge injection capacities compared to platinum.

PtIr is another material exhibiting a much higher charge injection capacity compared to platinum.

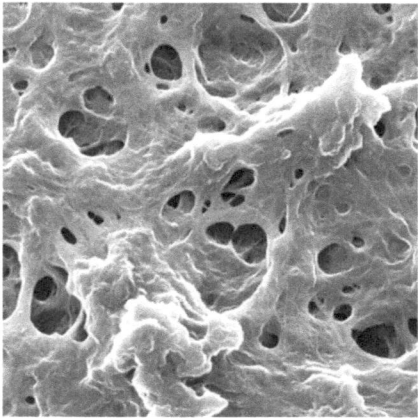

Fig. 6.2 Carbon nanotube structure of a PEDOT electrode, the picture is from Multi Channel Systems GmbH

Conducting polymers are considered to be advantageous alternatives. An example is poly(3,4-ethylenedioxythiophene) called PEDOT which is stable and biocompatible [33]. PEDOT has a charge injection capacity comparable to IrOx, which is about $2.3 \, mC/cm^2$ [7]. PEDOT can be combined with electrodeposited IrOx to enhance stability [25]. It is more stable than IrOx and TiN regarding chronic stimulation [7] and in contrary to IrOx does not need interpulse bias voltage for high charge injection capacity. S. Venkatraman et al. found out that PEDOT has 15 times more charge injection capacity compared to PtIr and electroplated IrOx (EIROF) using sub-millisecond current pulses and zero interpulse bias [30]. The major problem with PEDOT is its week adhesion to the underlying metal layers, which is the general problem with the polymers. Figure 6.2 shows the microscopic structure of PEDOT on an electrode.

In the following TiN and IrOx are investigated in more detail.

6.1   Titanium Nitride

6.1.1   TiN Material Characteristics: Safe Margins

The characteristics of TiN electrodes depend extensively on the fabrication technology, i.e. how porous and rough the electrode surface is made. For example the surface capacitance of the material was reported to be $35 \, mF/cm^2$ in [13], $0.5-1 \, mF/cm^2$ in [35], and $10 \, mF/cm^2$ in [24].

The limits for charge injection capacity also vary in the literature: The highest value of $23 \, mC/cm^2$ was reported in [9] (pulse length was 0.5 ms). In [32], while contradicting the results of [9], the safe charge limits were determined to be

$950\,\mu\text{C}/\text{cm}^2$ and $550\,\mu\text{C}/\text{cm}^2$ for 0.2 ms anodic and cathodic pulses, respectively. The electrodes were octagonal with an area of $4{,}000\,\mu\text{m}^2$. The charge injection capacity and the electrode capacitance depended on pulse length. Due to limits on the diffusion rates of charge carriers in the solution, higher frequency current pulses (i.e. current pulses with shorter length) correspond to a lower electrode-electrolyte interface capacitance. Longer pulse lengths naturally result in higher charge injection capacities also because more time is available for charge injection. In [35], the safe charge injection limit was determined to be in $2.2\text{--}3.5\,\text{mC}/\text{cm}^2$ range. The limits of safe charge injection were always determined based upon the assumed water window range in the study. In [5], using a cyclic voltammetry rate of $20\,\text{mV/s}$ and a smooth TiN film in PBS, a cathodic charge storage capacity (CSC_C) of only $250\,\mu\text{C}/\text{cm}^2$ was reported. CSC_C is essentially a measure of the total amount of charge available for a stimulation pulse (see Chap. 3).

The limits of water window are also different in the literature: The largest reported safe voltage window (water window) for TiN is -1 to $+1.2\,\text{V}$ (in PBS, versus Ag|AgCl, [35]). The water window reported in [5] is -0.9 to $+0.9\,\text{V}$, again versus Ag|AgCl. The reason for this discrepancy is the relatively qualitative approach used to determine the water window. Here, the cyclic voltammetry curve is investigated to recognize any oxidation/reduction boundaries. For example, in [35] the cyclic voltammetry vs. Ag|AgCl as in Fig. 6.3 was measured and the range of -1 to $+1.2\,\text{V}$ was determined. The boundaries are where the inflection points are located. The sharp increase for both the cathodic and anodic currents outside this range corresponds to the hydrolysis of water and gas evolution.

A precise investigation of the chemistry of thin film TiN electrodes was done in [14]. The thin films were between 20 and 300 nm thick. The boundaries in which no chemical reactions occur on TiN surface in 0.1 M phosphate buffer solution were determined to be between -0.3 and $+0.6\,\text{V}$ versus Ag|AgCl. This solution is different from PBS in that it contains no salt (NaCl) but higher phosphate concentration (0.1 M compared to 0.012 M for PBS).

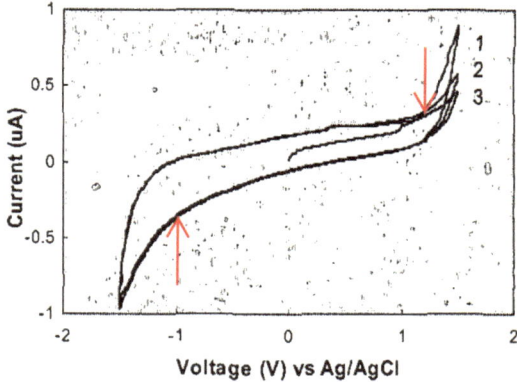

Fig. 6.3 Cyclic voltammogram of a TiN electrode at a potential scan rate of $100\,\text{mV/s}$, original picture (without the arrows) from [35], with permission

Table 6.1 A comparison between different TiN electrode parameters from different publications

Publication	Charge injection limit	Water window against Ag|AgCl	Interface capacitance
[13]	N.A.	N.A.	$35\,mF/cm^2$
[35]	$2.2–3.5\,mC/cm^2$	-1 to $+1.2$ V	$0.5–1\,mF/cm^2$
[24]	N.A.	N.A.	$10\,mF/cm^2$
[9]	$23\,mC/cm^2$	N.A.	N.A.
[5]	$1\,mC/cm^2$	-0.9 to $+0.9$ V	N.A.
[32]	$CSC_C = 250\,\mu C/cm^2$ $950\,\mu C/cm^2$ anodic $550\,\mu C/cm^2$ cathodic $0.2\,ms$ current pulses	-0.6 to 0.8 V	$1\,mF/cm^2$
[14]	N.A.	-0.3 to $+0.6$ V	N.A.

Table 6.1 lists the mentioned safe margins. The safe operation limits are typically smaller for cathodic polarity. Cathodic voltages are more harmful to TiN than the anodic ones [2].

In platinum, the charge injection capacity can be increased by imposing an anodic bias potential on the electrode between the current pulses [21, 27]. The same has not been reported for TiN.

As mentioned in Chap. 4, the most conservative approach to acquire long lifetime in chronic stimulation is limiting the electrode potential to water window. In order to determine the water window for TiN for chronic stimulation, biphasic triangular and rectangular voltage waveforms were generated by the manufactured signal generator and fed to 16 neighboring square electrodes in each experiment. While the waveforms had different amplitudes, they all had 0.3 ms cathodic and 0.5 ms anodic durations. After every biphasic pulse, the electrode was connected to ground via a 1 kΩ resistor for discharging. The tests ran until a major drop in the charge injection capacity was observed (electrode damage). When no damage occurred the test was stopped after 2 months. The electrode lifetime did not depend on the voltage waveform, but on the voltage limits. This confirms that the lifetime depends rather on the electrode potential amplitude limits than on the voltage drop on the Helmholtz capacitance, presumably because of the non-uniform electrode currents. A potential waveform outside ±1 V resulted in visible electrode damage (Fig. 6.4). For ±1 V, very little optical change and only 10 % decrease in charge injection and for ±0.5 V, no optical change or charge injection decrease was observed after 2 months [17]. The water window for this system of microelectrodes and a large TiN counter electrode was approximated to ±1 V. The charge injection capacity of TiN was measured to be $0.2\,mC/cm^2$ in the corresponding water window [17] (refer to Chap. 5 for the methodic). The water window of ±1 V extracted above is larger than the well known ±0.9 V from [5]. Actually the method of determining water window here is completely different from the literature. No silver-silver chloride reference electrode, but a two-electrode setup and a counter electrode made from the

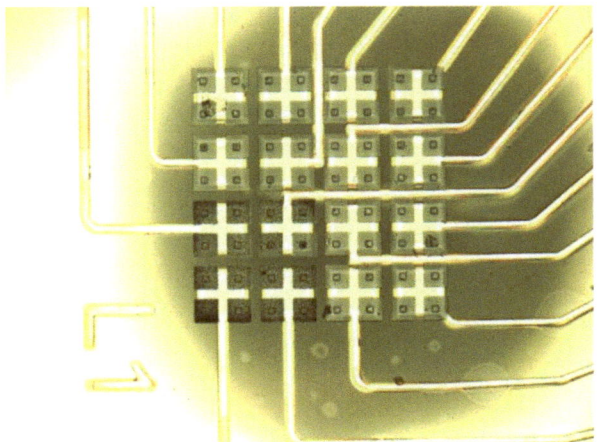

Fig. 6.4 TiN electrode oxidation after 1 week operation with triangular biphasic waveforms with ± 1.4 V amplitude. The active electrodes are on the *bottom left corner*. The others were not driven. Decrease in injected charge measured. Figure taken from [17], with permission ©2011 IEEE

same material as the microelectrodes is used here. This method is of a much larger practical significance, as in the real application (visual prosthesis) no reference electrode exists in the system.

6.1.2 Corrosion Properties of TiN

Reactions including corrosion occur even in distilled water around zero electrode potential, but they are very slow under these conditions. In the potential range from -200 to 10 mV against Ag|AgCl electrode, TiN reacts with water itself to form titanyl (TiO_2^{2+}) ions [11]. The half-reaction occurring at the TiN electrode is:

$$2TiN + 4H_2O \rightarrow 2TiO_2^{2+} + N_2 + 8H^+ + 12e^- \tag{6.1}$$

The products of this half-reaction are nitrogen gas and soluble ions. For electrode potentials from 10 mV to $+1.5$ V in NaCl solution, TiN dissolves in water to form Ti^{3+} ions.

Above 1.7 V, TiN is oxidized and thus passivated by formation of a titanium dioxide layer on it. The corrosion behavior of TiN has been compared to 12Kh18N10T steel using the method of potentiodynamic polarization curves in [11]. Figure 6.5 shows the corrosion rate (= corrosion current) of TiN as the working electrode versus voltage (vertical axis) for different media, the so called polarization curves. The counter electrode was a platinum plate and the reference electrode was a standard silver chloride Ag|AgCl electrode. The steel 12Kh18N10T (with alloying elements Mn, Cr, Ti) is used in stomatological practice. The experiment temperature

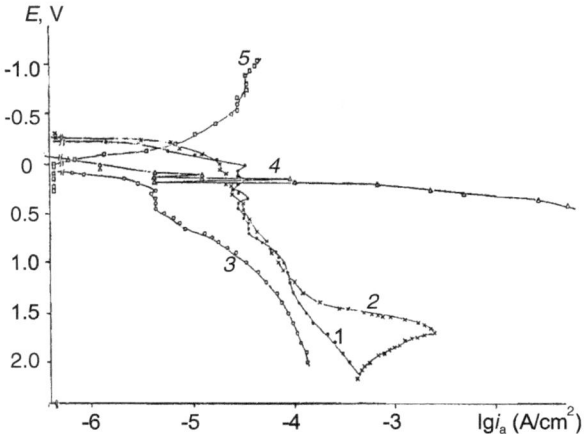

Fig. 6.5 Anodic polarization curves of TiN (*1*, *2*) and steel 12Kh18N10T (*3*, *4*) in distilled water (pH = 6.65; curves *1*, *3*) and 3 % NaCl solution (pH = 7.00; *2*, *4*); cathodic polarization curve of gold in distilled water (*5*), from [11], with permission

and the potential slope of the potentiostat were 37 °C and 0.5 mV/s, respectively. This study has been done to evaluate the corrosion behavior of different materials in the media of oral cavity. The cathodic polarization curve of gold was investigated because the steel or TiN prostheses may be found in the mouth along with gold crowns.

When in contact with other metals, pitting corrosion (galvanic corrosion) may occur with TiN films [15]. This happens for example, if the invasive medium (for example NaCl solution) penetrates the TiN layer due to its porosity and reaches the underlying metals. This corrosion happens also at zero electrode potential.

TiN coatings produced by physical vapor deposition (PVD) have a limited corrosion resistance due to their intrinsic porosity [15] and the presence of pores, pinholes and columnar structures [2]. When steel is used as substrate, a thicker TiN layer provides more resistance against corrosion [15]. This is probably because of the smaller number of defects in the film. The corrosion resistance can be enhanced by increasing the deposition temperature [2].

In [2] it is shown that TiN has a high cathodic corrosion current. According to polarization and cyclic voltammetry curves there, between voltages of −0.3 and −1.5 V for TiN coated electrode, the cathodic corrosion current is higher or comparable to the one from AISI 630 stainless steel. The reaction happening for negative voltages (smaller than −0.3 V) is:

$$2TiN + 4H_2O \rightarrow 2TiO_2 + N_2 + 4H_2 \tag{6.2}$$

This means that titanium dioxide forms also at negative electrode voltages. The investigated environment was a 0.1 M Na_2SO_4 solution with pHs between 6.2 and 13. For comparison, PBS solution has phosphate ions and its pH is 7.4.

The cathodic voltage may cause more damage to TiN than the anodic one [35]. Therefore, the safe boundaries for cathodic pulses are usually tighter than for the anodic ones. Moreover, shorter pulses impose tighter operation boundaries and the reversible reactions cannot be fully utilized with too short pulse lengths.

Anyway for TiN, even with an operation inside the safe margins, in chronic stimulation, corrosion still happens.

6.2   Iridium Oxide and Iridium

Iridium oxide has a superior charge injection capacity compared to TiN. Using 0.2 ms pulses and 4,000 μm^2 electrode area, a charge injection capacity of 4 mC/cm^2 has been measured for iridium oxide, compared to 550 μC/cm^2 for cathodic and 950 μC/cm^2 for anodic pulses in TiN in the same study. When compared to TiN, the large charge injection capacity of IrOx could allow for higher image resolution and lower power consumption in a retinal prosthesis. The larger charge injection capacity allows for smaller electrodes to be used to supply the same amount of charge [32].

6.2.1   Charge Transfer Mechanisms

The desire for microelectrodes with high charge injection capacities has led to development of electrode coatings based on faradaic charge injection mechanisms like iridium oxide [5]. As mentioned earlier, when the faradaic reactions are fast and the products do not leave the reaction site (e.g. no gases are produced), they can be reversed by current injection in an inverse direction. In contrast to titanium nitride, iridium oxide involves a hydrated oxide film on the metal surface and can inject charge into the electrolyte directly through electrons. Although this is a faradaic reaction involving reduction and oxidation between the Ir^{3+} and Ir^{4+} states of the oxide [5], its behavior resembles that of a capacitive reaction. This mechanism is called the "pseudo capacitive charge injection mechanism" [16]. In this case, the charge is saved and injected into the tissue from valence changes in a multivalent electrode coating that undergoes reversible redox reactions when a biphasic signal is fed into the electrode. These redox reactions include proton and hydroxyl ion transfers and have the following form [26]:

$$Ir^{3+}(OH)_3 + H_2O \leftrightarrow Ir^{4+}(OH)_4 + H^+ + e^- \qquad (6.3)$$

$$Ir^{3+}(OH)_3 + OH^- \leftrightarrow Ir^{4+}(OH)_4 + e^- \qquad (6.4)$$

A positive inter-pulse bias voltage between 0.4 and 0.8 V versus Ag|AgCl can increase the charge injection capacity of iridium oxide up to as high as three times [5]. This bias voltage polarizes the iridium oxide from a mixed Ir^{3+}/Ir^{4+} valence state to the Ir^{4+} valence state. The Ir^{4+} valence state is considerably more conducting and makes available more Ir^{4+} for reduction during cathodic pulse [5]. An inter-pulse potential of 0.7 V versus Ag|AgCl was applied in [28], while in [1] this was 0.8 V versus SCE, where only cathodic current pulses were injected. In practice applying a positive inter-pulse offset to the iridium oxide electrode must be done with caution. The neural prosthetic systems usually include stimulation and counter electrodes, and no reference electrode which would control the solution potential. A platinum reference electrode was used for chronical stimulation for over 4 years in one case [5]. Platinum builds a stable potential of around 0 V versus Ag|AgCl in vivo [5].

Another reason for higher charge injection capacity with a positive inter-pulse offset voltage is presumably a higher double layer capacitance for more positive electrode potentials. At higher potentials the higher electric field absorbs the oppositely loaded ions towards the electrode surface and therefore the double layer thickness reduces.

Impedance spectroscopy measurements with a large iridium counter electrode as the reference (two-electrode structure) and with a DC voltage on the disk shaped iridium microelectrodes showed a reduction in the impedance amplitude values and the slope over frequency. This indicates an increase in the interface capacitance when a bias voltage exists on the electrode. As long as the DC voltage is inside the water window, no irreversible reactions may occur. As illustrated in Fig. 6.6, for DC voltages in the ranges $-0.6\,V \rightarrow -0.4\,V$ and $0.4\,V \rightarrow 0.5\,V$ versus OCP a decrease in the impedance amplitude spectra specially for lower frequencies is visible. To illustrate the 3D diagram better, the frequency axis is labeled from higher to lower frequencies.

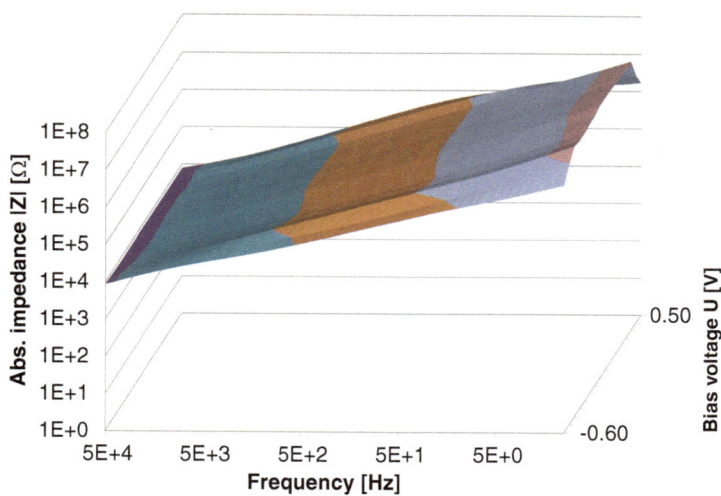

Fig. 6.6 3D presentation of the impedance amplitude spectra for different electrode bias voltages

Asymmetric charge balanced waveforms in which the anodic pulse is delivered at a lower current but a longer pulse length compared to the cathodic one were found to allow higher values of anodic bias voltages, thus maximizing the iridium oxide charge injection capacity [28].

6.2.2 Manufacturing Methods

Iridium oxide electrodes can be classified into four types based on the manufacturing method:

- AIROF (Activated Iridium Oxide Film)
- SIROF (Sputtered Iridium Oxide Film)
- TIROF (Thermally prepared Iridium Oxide Film)
- EIROF (Electrodeposited Iridium Oxide Film)

The most prevalent ones are AIROF and SIROF.

For manufacturing AIROF, an iridium electrode is inserted into an acidic or buffer electrolyte and electrically activated. Investigations have shown that AIROF electrodes are very good in biocompatibility, good in lifetime but bad in reproducibility.

Activating iridium means oxidizing it to increase the amount of charge injection capacity. The oxidization reactions occur at positive voltages outside water window (≥ 0.8 V versus Ag|AgCl). Hydrogen molecules resulting from the reaction should have enough time to diffuse away from the electrode surface or escape the electrode surface as gas bubbles if larger amounts is produced, thus slowly varying waveforms are preferred. The resulting iridium oxide layer has a much larger volume compared to the original iridium layer. For example, activating a $160\,\text{Å}$ thick iridium layer results in iridium oxide with a thickness of $1{,}300\,\text{Å}$ after complete oxidization [12]. Weiland et al. [31] activated pure iridium by a 0.5 Hz, 50 % duty cycle square wave with the voltage amplitudes of -0.7 V and $+0.8$ V versus saturated calomel electrode (SCE) using a potentiostat. Lee et al. [12] used a cyclic ramp voltage between 0 V and $+1.4$ V versus standard hydrogen electrode (SHE) with a rate of 100 mV/s for activation. Another activation method was suggested by Robblee and Rose [20] in which 500 cycles of a periodic triangular voltage varying between -0.7 V and $+1.2$ V against Ag|AgCl with 100 mV/s is put on the electrodes.

This method was used in the experiments here with a difference. As there is no reference electrode in the final product (subretinal prosthesis) it was tried to activate iridium with considering a large iridium counter electrode as potential reference. As a single standard reduction potential cannot be defined for an iridium electrode no proper voltage range could be derived for electrode activation by theoretical means. Therefore, this method had to be tested again for this special case. In [18] a 120 % increase in the charge injection capacity of the $50 \times 50\,\mu\text{m}$ square electrodes using this method was reported. Charge injection capacity was calculated by using a rectangular electrode voltage (cathodic/anodic pulse duration

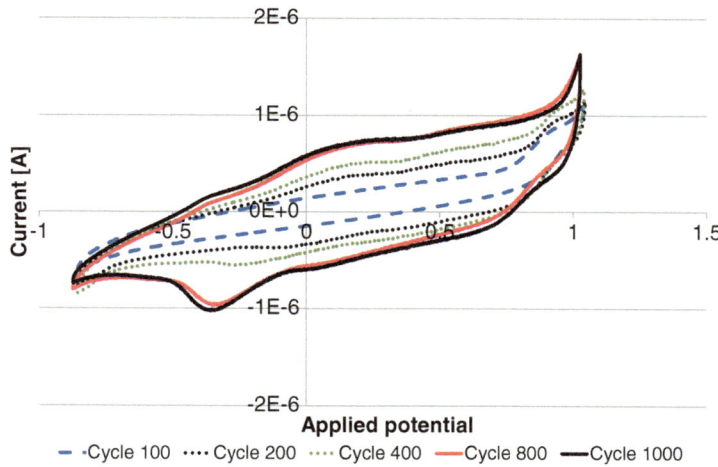

Fig. 6.7 Cyclic voltammetry curves of ten parallel electrodes of MEA 2 for different activation levels, working versus counter electrode voltage range is between -0.7 V $\rightarrow$ $+1.2$ V versus OCP which was -175 mV here

$= 0.3$ ms/0.5 ms) limited to the -0.6 V $\rightarrow$ $+0.8$ V voltage range versus the iridium counter electrode (see Sect. 5.3). Iridium can also be activated with faster voltage waveforms but no activation was observed with a voltage waveform similar to the one used by Weiland et al. but having a frequency of 2 Hz instead of 0.5 Hz and no Ag|AgCl reference electrode even after several days. This shows that the oxidization reaction kinetics for iridium is too slow to happen by a 2 Hz pulse at -0.7 V $\rightarrow$ $+0.8$ V with iridium as the counter electrode. When higher positive voltages were used ($+1.2$ V), iridium could be activated after 24 h.

The disc shaped iridium electrodes were activated. Cyclic voltammetry function of the potentiostat was used to generate the Robblee waveform. The potentiostat was simultaneously measuring the resulting current flowing from ten parallel connected electrodes into the counter electrode. Figure 6.7 shows the cyclic voltammetry measurement results of several electrodes from MEA 2 connected in parallel to the potentiostat after various numbers of activation cycles. For MEA 2, 1,500 activation cycles were used to investigate the effect of continuing activation beyond the number of cycles suggested by Robblee. In every cycle, some charge is stored irreversibly in the oxide layer. The charge transferred by the electrodes into the solution in each cycle is equal to the area inside the CV curve. The microelectrode voltage range covers 1.9 V, so it is certainly outside the water window for iridium (-0.6 V $\rightarrow$ $+0.8$ V vs. Ag|AgCL) which covers 1.4 V. Therefore, the transferred charge is not equal to the recoverable stored charge corresponding to a reversible redox reaction. After 800 cycles the area enclosed by the CV curve remains almost the same, therefore Fig. 6.7 contains measurement information of only the first 1,000 cycles. No considerable increase in the transferred charge is observable above 500 cycles for both MEAs, as predicted by the Robblee method.

Table 6.2 Average charge injection capacities of MEA 1 and MEA 2 electrodes before activation

	MEA1 1	MEA1 2	MEA 2
Charge injection capacity Q_{inj} (mC/cm^2)	0.39	0.74	0.47

Table 6.3 Average charge injection capacity of ten electrodes from MEA 1 and ten electrodes from MEA 2 for different activation levels

MEA 1	Q_{inj} (mC/cm^2)	MEA 2	Q_{inj} (mC/cm^2)
Before activation	0.6		0.5
After 100 cycles	1.1		0.7
After 200 cycles	3.3		3.5
After 300 cycles	3.8		4.0
After 400 cycles	4.3		x
After 500 cycles	4.5		4.0
After 1,500 cycles	x		4.5

Before activation the charge injection capacity of the disc electrodes was measured by the method explained in Sect. 5.3. Outliers were neglected. The measurement error was estimated to be under 6 %. Table 6.2 shows the average results. For MEA 1 two distinct groups were observed, with a third of the electrodes having the higher charge injection capacity.

Table 6.3 shows the charge injection capacities at different activation levels. The charge injection capacity for both MEAs could be increased to 4.5 mC/cm^2. The highest increase occurs between cycle numbers 100 and 200.

A photograph of a MEA 2 activated electrode after 1,500 cycles is illustrated in Fig. 6.8. The neighboring three electrodes are not activated. The activated electrode has a darker color due to the built oxide layer. The surface of the activated color is not uniformly colored. The periphery is darker while the middle is lighter. This corresponds to higher current levels resulting in more oxidation reactions and consequently more activation at the periphery compared to the center. As the electrode voltage turns positive enough to cause irreversible reactions, the surface Helmholtz capacitance breaks down. As a result, the structure resembles to a disk electrode in contact with a conductive solution. The outcome is the non-uniform electrode current distribution as illustrated previously in Fig. 4.2.

It is beneficial if the prosthetic device would provide the ability to activate the electrodes if iridium electrodes are fabricated. Activating iridium electrodes is possible in the stimulator chip in [22]: A special mode can be activated to connect the electrodes continuously to ground. The counter electrode can be swept by a triangular voltage opposite in polarity to the Robblee waveform. The activation current per electrode is at most a few hundred nanoamperes (Fig. 6.7) which can be easily supported by a transistor switch per electrode without considerable voltage drop on the switch.

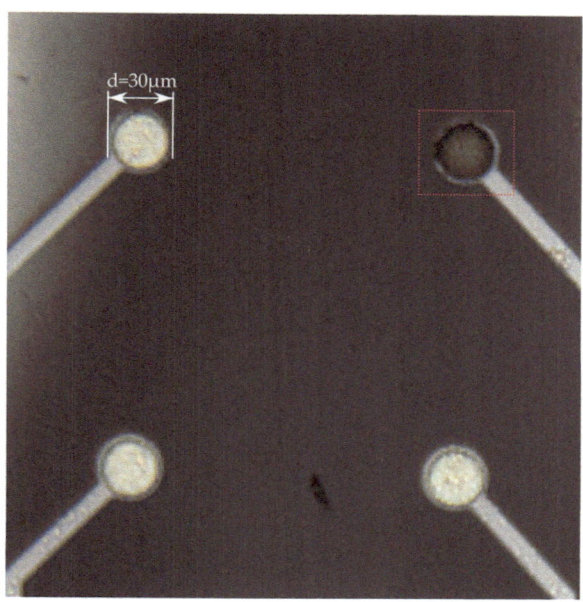

Fig. 6.8 Four electrodes from MEA 2. The activated electrode is marked, picture from [10]

Much better in reproducibility, mechanical properties and also very good in biocompatibility are the SIROF electrodes. For the production of SIROF, iridium oxide is sputtered reactively on platinum or gold. An iridium target as well as a reactive gaseous mixture of argon and oxygen in a 1.45:1 ratio with a pressure of 0.012 mbar is applied. SIROF has a smaller charge injection capacity compared to AIROF.

Many challenges exist for the manufacturing of TIROF or EIROF electrodes. They are both expensive. For the production of TIROF temperatures up to 550 °C is needed which can damage polyimide layers. Polyimide is a polymer used extensively in implant systems for isolating the devices from water. For the fabrication of EIROF electrodes the electrolyte must have a pH value of exactly 10.5. Even small fluctuations of pH deteriorate the reproducibility of EIROF electrodes.

Although iridium oxide has a higher charge injection capacity than iridium, metallic iridium can also be applied as an electrode material. Table 6.4 lists a comparison between the properties of iridium, AIROF and SIROF. As seen in this table, iridium has some superior properties compared to both AIROF and SIROF, although they both have the advantage of providing a higher charge injection capacity.

Table 6.4 A comparison between the properties of iridium, AIROF and SIROF ($++$ very good; $+$ good; $-$ bad) [18]

Material	Mechanical properties	Biocompat- ibility	Long-term stability	Reproduc- ibility
Iridium	$++$	$++$	$++$	$++$
AIROF	$+$	$++$	$+$	$-$
SIROF	$++$	$++$	$+$	$++$

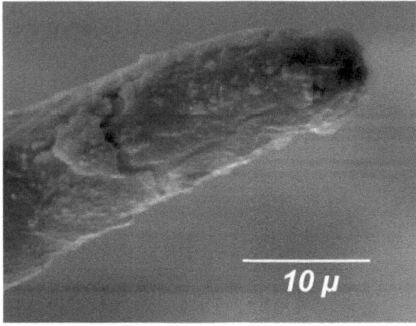

Fig. 6.9 Scanning electron microscope photograph of an AIROF electrode showing delamination due to cathodic voltage excursions below -0.6 V against Ag|AgCl. This damage is irreversible and deteriorates the charge injection capacity of the electrode considerably. From [28], with permission ©2004 IEEE

6.2.3 Safe Operation Margins

The safe operation window ($=$water window) for iridium oxide (IrOx) is -0.6 V $\rightarrow$ $+0.8$ V versus Ag|AgCl [28, 32]. Outside this range electrode damage and solution pH change are possible. For cathodic excursions below -0.6 V versus Ag|AgCl delamination of AIROF may occur which is not reversible and deteriorates the electrode properties considerably (Fig. 6.9). This delamination can be identified by a sharp anodic discontinuity of the cyclic voltammetry plot as shown in Fig. 6.10 [28].

It is better to consider the -0.6 and $+0.8$ V versus Ag|AgCl potential boundaries for the electrode potential without subtracting the $I \cdot R$ drop on the electrode access resistance ($=$ access voltage). It was observed that when the electrode potential subtracted by the access voltage is used as the variable to be limited inside the water window, electrodes were damaged. This is because of the non-uniformity of the current distribution on the electrode surface and because the maximum potential excursions are not constant over the electrode geometry [28].

The charge injection capacity of iridium oxide was evaluated as $4\,\mathrm{m\,C/cm^2}$ in [32]. Troyk et al. have developed a simple but effective current cutback method to retain the electrode potential inside the water window. In this method, the supply voltages of the electrode driver current sources are set to the water window voltage boundaries. In this way, with only a modest decrease in charge injection, the

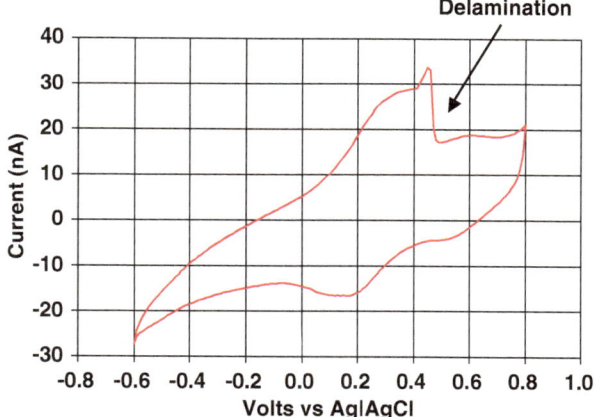

Fig. 6.10 Cyclic voltammetry curve providing evidence of AIROF delamination, from [28], with permission ©2004 IEEE

Table 6.5 Cathodic charge injection limits of AIROF electrode as a function of frequency and pulse width for an interpulse bias voltage of +0.7 V [6]

	Pulse width	
Frequency (Hz)	0.2 ms	0.4 ms
20	$3.4\,\text{mC/cm}^2$	$3.9\,\text{mC/cm}^2$
50	$2.9\,\text{mC/cm}^2$	$3.8\,\text{mC/cm}^2$
100	$2.1\,\text{mC/cm}^2$	$3.2\,\text{mC/cm}^2$

electrode is kept inside the $-0.6\,\text{V} \rightarrow +0.8\,\text{V}$ voltage range [28]. The cathodic charge injection capacity they measured for a $1{,}000\,\mu\text{m}^2$ electrode and a cathodic pulse length of $300\,\mu\text{s}$ was $1.86\,\text{m C/cm}^2$. To achieve this in hardware, the positive supply of the output driver was set to $+0.7\,\text{V}$, so the anodic pulse injection transistor injects current into the electrode till the electrode potential reaches $+0.7\,\text{V}$. The electrode was maintained at $+0.7\,\text{V}$ anodic bias during the interpulse interval, in order to achieve a higher charge injection capacity.

Table 6.5 lists the charge injection capacity of AIROF for different frequencies according to Cogan et al. [6]. For higher frequencies the charge injection capacity decreased more for shorter pulse widths compared to longer ones.

Xenia Beebe et al. evaluated the maximum charge injection capacity of activated iridium wire electrodes in bicarbonate buffered saline as $2.1\,\text{m C/cm}^2$ and $1.0\,\text{m C/cm}^2$ for anodic-first and cathodic-first, $0.2\,\text{ms}$ charge balanced biphasic current pulses, respectively [1]. Bicarbonate buffered saline has a pH between 7.35 and 7.45 (similar to the human blood plasma) and is comparable to PBS with a pH value of 7.4. The counter electrode was an iridium foil. The reference electrode was a saturated calomel electrode. Cyclic voltammetry at $100\,\text{mV/s}$ revealed a water window of $-0.6\,\text{V} \rightarrow +0.8\,\text{V}$, the same as versus Ag|AgCl.

As in the subretinal stimulation structure no reference electrode is available, the above ranges are not applicable, because the solution potential is not controlled by a reference electrode. Furthermore, if any faradaic reactions occur, the solution potential and therefore the water window depend on the relative total area of the active working (stimulation) electrodes to the area of the counter electrode. A very large counter electrode has a large interface double layer capacitance, therefore its polarization (i.e. the deviation from the unknown equilibrium electrode potential) can be neglected for the currents emerging from the much smaller working electrodes. Consequently, instead of being set by a reference electrode, the solution potential is set by the electrode potential of the counter electrode. Therefore, in order to determine the water window for this arrangement, the large iridium counter electrode was used as the reference and put on the ground.

In the first approach, lifetime tests for iridium microelectrodes were run. Groups of 4 or 16 neighboring electrodes were connected to the signal generator discussed in Chap. 5. Biphasic rectangular voltages of a cathodic pulse length of 0.3 ms, anodic pulse length of 0.5 ms and period of 3 ms were used. Rectangular voltage pulses result in the maximum charge injection for the given potential limits [17]. Figure 6.11 shows the results. It is seen here that when the electrode potential is limited to the -0.6 V $\rightarrow$ $+0.8$ V range, no drop in the electrode charge injection is observed even after 2 months.

According to Fig. 6.11 the charge injection capacity of iridium is about 0.5 mC/cm^2 in the -0.6 V $\rightarrow$ $+0.8$ V range. The charge injection dropped for an electrode potential waveform limited in the $\pm$ 1 V range. So the water window for the electrode arrangement composed of four adjacent 50×50 µm electrodes and a much larger counter electrode (0.5 cm^2) is somewhere between -0.6 V and $+0.8$ V and $\pm$ 1 V ranges. Fewer adjacent active electrodes result in more charge injection for a certain biphasic pulse voltage amplitude at the beginning (look at the curve corresponding to ± 2 V), but the charge injection drops faster. This has two reasons:

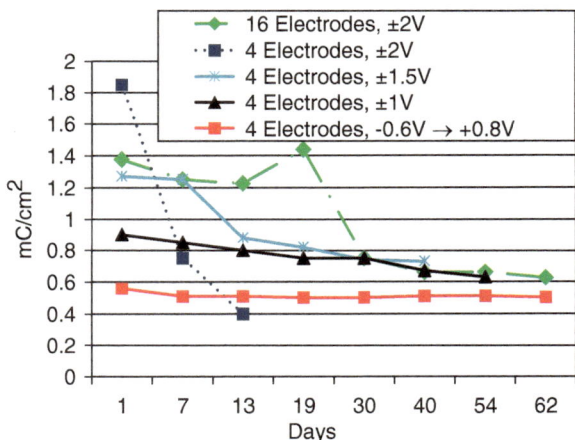

Fig. 6.11 Maximum charge injection over time for different electrode potential boundaries [19] ©2012 IEEE

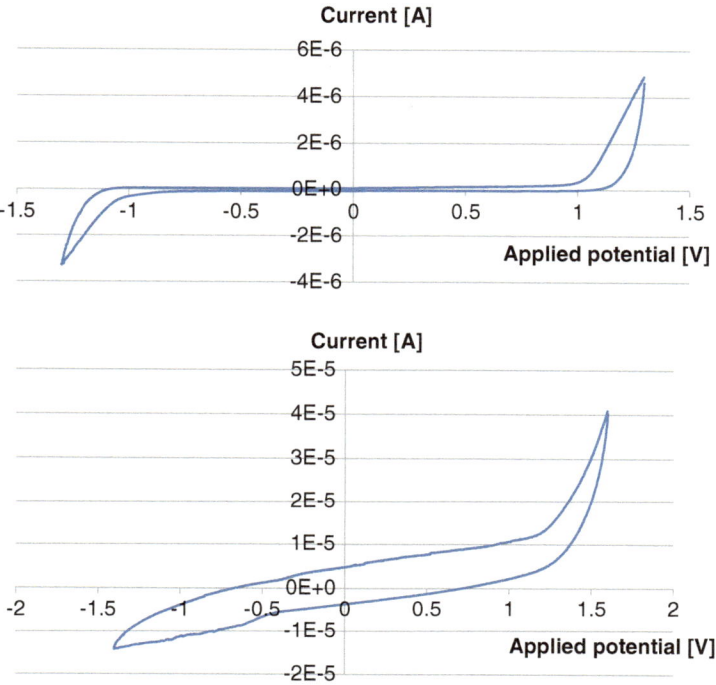

Fig. 6.12 *Upper picture* illustrates CV curve of four adjacent square iridium electrodes against the counter electrode. Voltage range is ±1.3 V versus the counter electrode. *Lower picture* illustrates CV curve of 64 adjacent electrodes against the counter electrode. Voltage range is −1.4 to 1.6 V versus the counter electrode

1. For more electrodes, the assumption of negligible total working electrodes area is not valid any more. The voltage drop on the counter electrode due to charge injection (the polarization of the counter electrode) is not negligible any more. As the voltage drop between the working and the counter electrode is distributed on both electrodes' interface capacitances, more voltage difference is needed to cause the same amount of faradaic reactions to occur. In other words, as the counter electrode must carry more faradaic current, the overpotential needed to inject this current into the counter electrode is higher. Therefore, for a higher number of active working electrodes, the water window is wider. Figure 6.12 shows the CV curve one time for only four adjacent electrodes of an iridium MEA (shown in Fig. 5.2) and the other time for 64 electrodes. For four electrodes the water window is almost a symmetrical ±1 V, as defined by the inflection points (see Fig. 6.3 for comparison). For 64 electrodes the water window cannot be wholly detected in the applied CV range: The negative boundary lies below −1.4 V and the positive is at around +1.2 V.

2. When the number of active electrodes is smaller, the overall electrical field distribution is more compact. Therefore, the potential difference between the electrode metal and the immediate surrounding solution, i.e. the Helmholtz

capacitor voltage drop at the stimulation electrodes, is higher. This causes a faster deterioration. A detailed analysis on electrical field distribution around electrodes is presented in [23].

References

1. Beebe X, Rose TL (1988) Charge injection limits of activated iridium oxide electrodes with 0.2 ms pulses in bicarbonate buffered saline (neurological stimulation application). Biomedical Engineering, IEEE Transactions on 35(6):494–495, DOI 10.1109/10.2122
2. Bellanger G, Rameau JJ (1995) Corrosion of titanium nitride deposits on AISI 630 stainless steel used in radioactive water with and without chloride at pH 11. Electrochimica Acta 40(15):2519–2532, DOI 10.1016/0013-4686(94)00326-V, URL http://www.sciencedirect.com/science/article/pii/001346869400326V
3. Boretius T, Jurzinsky T, Koehler C, Kerzenmacher S, Hillebrecht H, Stieglitz T (2011) High-porous platinum electrodes for functional electrical stimulation. In: Engineering in Medicine and Biology Society,EMBC, 2011 Annual International Conference of the IEEE, pp 5404–5407, DOI 10.1109/IEMBS.2011.6091336
4. Brummer SB, Robblee LS, Hambrecht FT (1983) Criteria for selecting electrodes for electrical stimulation: Theoretical and practical considerations. Annals of the New York Academy of Sciences 405(1):159–171, DOI 10.1111/j.1749-6632.1983.tb31628.x, URL http://dx.doi.org/10.1111/j.1749-6632.1983.tb31628.x
5. Cogan SF (2008) Neural stimulation and recording electrodes. Tech. rep., EIC Laboratories
6. Cogan SF, Troyk PR, Ehrlich J, Plante TD (2005) In vitro comparison of the charge-injection limits of activated iridium oxide (AIROF) and platinum-iridium microelectrodes. Biomedical Engineering, IEEE Transactions on 52(9):1612–1614, DOI 10.1109/TBME.2005.851503
7. Cui XT, Zhou DD (2007) Poly (3,4-ethylenedioxythiophene) for chronic neural stimulation. Neural Systems and Rehabilitation Engineering, IEEE Transactions on 15(4):502–508, DOI 10.1109/TNSRE.2007.909811
8. Hassler C, Guy J, Nietzschmann M, Staiger JF, Stieglitz T (2011) Chronic intracortical implantation of saccharose-coated flexible shaft electrodes into the cortex of rats. In: Engineering in Medicine and Biology Society,EMBC, 2011 Annual International Conference of the IEEE, pp 644–647, DOI 10.1109/IEMBS.2011.6090143
9. Janders M, Egert U, Stelzle M, Nisch W (1996) Novel thin film titanium nitride microelectrodes with excellent charge transfer capability for cell stimulation and sensing applications. In: Engineering in Medicine and Biology Society, 1996. Bridging Disciplines for Biomedicine. Proceedings of the 18th Annual International Conference of the IEEE, vol 1, pp 245–247 vol. 1, DOI 10.1109/IEMBS.1996.656936
10. Kaim H (2013) Charakterisierung und elektrische Ansteuerung von Stimulations-Elektroden. Diplomarbeit, University of Ulm
11. Lavrenko VA, Shvets VA, Makarenko GN (2001) Comparative study of the chemical resistance of titanium nitride and stainless steel in media of the oral cavity. Powder Metallurgy and Metal Ceramics 40:630–636, URL http://dx.doi.org/10.1023/A:1015296323497, 10.1023/A:1015296323497
12. Lee IS (2004) Neural cells on iridium oxide. Key Engineering Materials 254–256:805–808
13. Norlin A, Pan J, Leygraf C (2002) Investigation of interfacial capacitance of Pt, Ti and TiN coated electrodes by electrochemical impedance spectroscopy. Biomol Eng 19(2–6):67–71, URL http://www.biomedsearch.com/nih/Investigation-interfacial-capacitance-Pt-Ti/12202164.html

14. Nunes Kirchner C, Hallmeier KH, Szargan R, Raschke T, Radehaus C, Wittstock G (2007) Evaluation of thin film titanium nitride electrodes for electroanalytical applications. Electroanalysis 19(10):1023–1031, DOI 10.1002/elan.200703832, URL http://dx.doi.org/10.1002/elan.200703832

15. Perillo PM (2006) Corrosion behavior of coatings of titanium nitride and titanium-titanium nitride on steel substrates. CORROSION 62

16. Poppendieck W (2010) Untersuchungen zum Einsatz neuer Elektrodenmaterialien: Und deren Evaluation als Reiz- und Ableitelektrode. Südwestdeutscher Verlag, URL http://books.google.de/books?id=Z1xnRwAACAAJ

17. Pour Aryan N, Asad M, Brendler C, Kibbel S, Heusel G, Rothermel A (2011) In vitro study of titanium nitride electrodes for neural stimulation. In: Engineering in Medicine and Biology Society,EMBC, 2011 Annual International Conference of the IEEE, pp 2866–2869, DOI 10.1109/IEMBS.2011.6090791

18. Pour Aryan N, Brendler C, Rieger V, Kibbel S, Harscher A, Heusel G, Rothermel A (2012a) A comparison of TiN, iridium and iridium oxide stimulating electrodes for neural stimulation. In: International Association of Science and Technology for Development,BioMed, 2012 Annual International Conference

19. Pour Aryan N, Brendler C, Rieger V, Schleehauf S, Heusel G, Rothermel A (2012b) In vitro study of iridium electrodes for neural stimulation. In: Engineering in Medicine and Biology Society,EMBC, 2012 Annual International Conference of the IEEE

20. Robblee LS, Rose TL (1990) Electrochemical Guidelines for Selection of Protocols and Electrode Materials for Neural Stimulation. In Neural Prostheses (Hrsg.: Agnew, W.F.; McCreery, D.B.), Prentice Hall, Englewood Cliffs, New Jersey, S. 25–66

21. Rose TL, Robblee LS (1990) Electrical stimulation with Pt electrodes. VIII. Electrochemically safe charge injection limits with 0.2 ms pulses (neuronal application). Biomedical Engineering, IEEE Transactions on 37(11):1118–1120, DOI 10.1109/10.61038

22. Rothermel A, Liu L, Aryan NP, Fischer M, Wünschmann J, Kibbel S, Harscher A (2009) A CMOS chip with active pixel array and specific test features for subretinal implantation. IEEE Journal of Solid-State Circuits 44(1):290–299

23. Rubinstein JT, Spelman FA, Soma M, Suesserman MF (1987) Current density profiles of surface mounted and recessed electrodes for neural prostheses. Biomedical Engineering, IEEE Transactions on BME-34(11):864–875, DOI 10.1109/TBME.1987.326007

24. Schaldach M, Hubmann M, Weikl A, Hardt R (1990) Sputter-deposited TiN electrode coatings for superior sensing and pacing performance. Pacing and Clinical Electrophysiology 13(12):1891–1895, DOI 10.1111/j.1540-8159.1990.tb06911.x, URL http://dx.doi.org/10.1111/j.1540-8159.1990.tb06911.x

25. Shanmugasundaram B, Gluckman BJ (2011) Micro-reaction chamber electrodes for neural stimulation and recording. In: Engineering in Medicine and Biology Society,EMBC, 2011 Annual International Conference of the IEEE, pp 656–659, DOI 10.1109/IEMBS.2011.6090146

26. Stieglitz T (2004) Materials for stimulation and recording. Tech. rep., Neural Prosthetics Group, Fraunhofer Institute for Biomedical Engineering

27. Terasawa Y, Tashiro H, Uehara A, Saitoh T, Ozawa M, Tokuda T, Ohta J (2006) The development of a multichannel electrode array for retinal prostheses. Journal of Artificial Organs 9:263–266, URL http://dx.doi.org/10.1007/s10047-006-0352-1, 10.1007/s10047-006-0352-1

28. Troyk PR, Detlefsen DE, Cogan SF, Ehrlich J, Bak M, McCreery DB, Bullara L, Schmidt E (2004) "Safe" charge-injection waveforms for iridium oxide (AIROF) microelectrodes. In: Engineering in Medicine and Biology Society, 2004. IEMBS '04. 26th Annual International Conference of the IEEE, vol 2, pp 4141–4144, DOI 10.1109/IEMBS.2004.1404155

29. Vanhoestenberghe A, Donaldson N, Lovell N, Suaning G (2008) Hermetic encapsulation of an implantable vision prosthesis - combining implant fabrication philosophies. In: IFESS 2008 - from movement to mind, URL http://discovery.ucl.ac.uk/1318417/

30. Venkatraman S, Hendricks J, King Z, Sereno A, Richardson-Burns S, Martin D, Carmena J (2011) In vitro and in vivo evaluation of PEDOT microelectrodes for neural stimulation and recording. Neural Systems and Rehabilitation Engineering, IEEE Transactions on 19(3):307–316, DOI 10.1109/TNSRE.2011.2109399

31. Weiland JD, Anderson DJ (2000) Chronic neural stimulation with thin-film, iridium oxide electrodes. Biomedical Engineering, IEEE Transactions on 47(7):911–918, DOI 10.1109/10.846685

32. Weiland JD, Anderson DJ, Humayun MS (2002) In vitro electrical properties for iridium oxide versus titanium nitride stimulating electrodes. Biomedical Engineering, IEEE Transactions on 49(12):1574–1579, DOI 10.1109/TBME.2002.805487

33. Wilks SJ, Woolley AJ, Ouyang L, Martin DC, Otto KJ (2011) In vivo polymerization of poly (3,4-ethylenedioxythiophene) (PEDOT) in rodent cerebral cortex. In: Engineering in Medicine and Biology Society,EMBC, 2011 Annual International Conference of the IEEE, pp 5412–5415, DOI 10.1109/IEMBS.2011.6091338

34. Winkin N, Mokwa W (2012) Flexible multi-electrode array with integrated bendable CMOS-Chip for implantable systems. In: Engineering in Medicine and Biology Society,EMBC, 2012 Annual International Conference of the IEEE

35. Zhou DM, Greenberg RJ (2003) Electrochemical characterization of titanium nitride microelectrode arrays for charge-injection applications. In: Engineering in Medicine and Biology Society, 2003. Proceedings of the 25th Annual International Conference of the IEEE, vol 2, pp 1964–1967 Vol. 2, DOI 10.1109/IEMBS.2003.1279831

Chapter 7
The Effect of the Counter Electrode on Stimulation Electrode Lifetime

In electrostimulation, if redox reactions occur, they always happen in two distinct but simultaneous oxidation and reduction half-reaction groups at anode and cathode, which are the working and the counter electrodes depending on the injected signal polarity. A half-reaction cannot happen without the occurrence of its complementary opposite counterpart. Therefore, the size and the material of the counter electrode affects the water window.

In the case where the counter (return) electrode is small and located near the working (stimulation) electrode, like the structure used in the photovoltaic subretinal implant reported in [1] (see Fig. 7.1), the counter electrode has an interface capacitance comparable to that of the stimulating electrode. The working versus counter electrode voltage drop is then shared by the two series interface capacitances of the electrodes in comparable proportions. Therefore, higher voltages are allowable for the same amount of faradaic currents, meaning the water window is wider. This was implicitly confirmed with the experiments in last chapter, where a higher number of active working electrodes led to a larger water window and lower DC currents flowing for the same applied electrode potential amplitudes (see Fig. 6.12).

In the monopolar stimulation arrangement investigated more precisely here, where the counter electrode is much larger than a single stimulation electrode and is located at a relatively distant position, the water window depends on the number of active electrodes as was shown in Fig. 6.12. The higher the number of the stimulating electrodes, the wider the water window.

© The Author(s) 2015
N. Pour Aryan et al., *Stimulation and Recording Electrodes for Neural Prostheses*,
SpringerBriefs in Electrical and Computer Engineering 78,
DOI 10.1007/978-3-319-10052-4_7

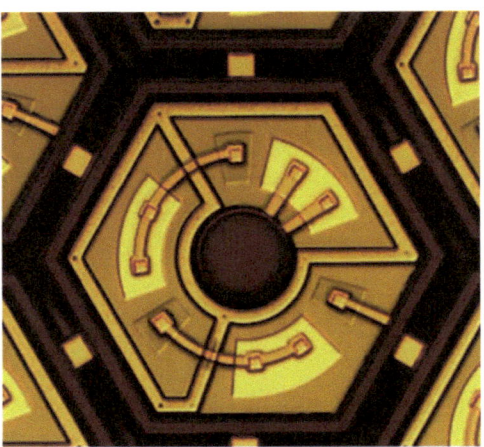

Fig. 7.1 The working and the counter electrode of one stimulating pixel in the subretinal implant of [1], the working electrode is the disk in the *middle* and the counter electrode is the hexagonal ring at periphery, both in *dark brown*, picture from [1], with permission

7.1   The Effect of Counter Electrode Material on Faradaic Reactions During Electrostimulation

Even when few electrodes are active and therefore the total area of the working electrodes is negligible compared to the counter electrode, with an area of $0.5 \, cm^2$ here, the water window and the DC (faradaic) currents flowing still depend on the counter electrode material. Using four square $50 \times 50 \, \mu m$ iridium microelectrodes and three different counter electrode materials, three CV curves were measured while always the same four microelectrodes were driven. The results are illustrated in Fig. 7.2. The inflection points in the forward positive and forward negative scans define the water window (see Fig. 6.3 for comparison). Therefore, water window for the four adjacent electrodes can be evaluated as almost ± 1 V for iridium and gold counter electrodes and an asymmetrical range of about -1.2 to $+0.9$ V with TiN as counter electrode material. Furthermore, the faradaic currents are lower for gold as the counter electrode at the CV voltage boundaries which are located outside the water window. TiN counter electrode causes relatively large oxidation faradaic currents at the iridium stimulation electrodes when the corresponding higher limit of the water window is exceeded. Although for the special case of iridium, oxidation currents are not necessarily harmful to the electrodes as iridium oxide is also a conducting material, tissue damage is resulted because of gas evolution and pH change and thus these currents must be avoided. Furthermore, oxidation currents also generally damage electrodes when other materials are used.

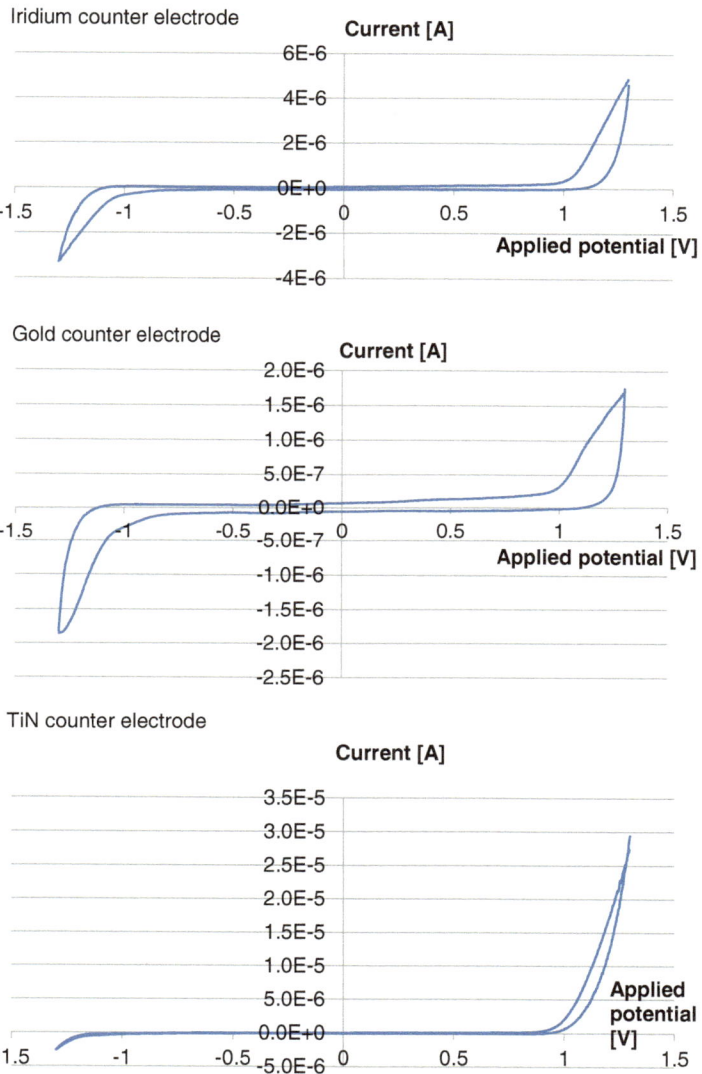

Fig. 7.2 CV curve of four iridium electrodes against an iridium counter electrode (*upper picture*), against gild counter electrode (*middle picture*), and against TiN counter electrode (*lower picture*), voltage range is ±1.3 V versus the counter electrode

7.2 The Effect of Counter Electrode Material on Galvanic Corrosion

As explained before, for charge balancing the working electrodes are either connected directly to the counter electrode after the stimulation pulse, or they are kept at the same potential by means of active circuitry. In both cases a small galvanic

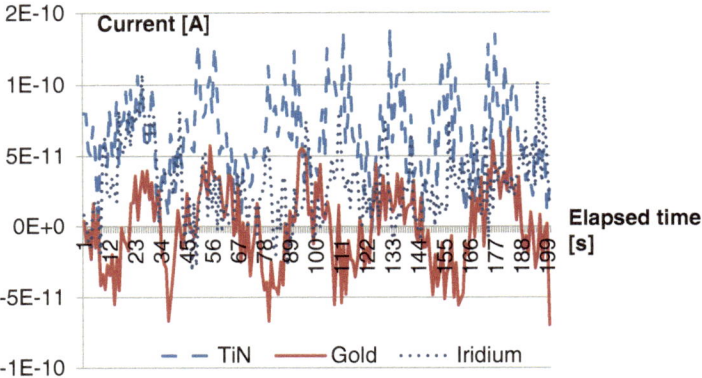

Fig. 7.3 Galvanic corrosion current for different counter electrode materials

corrosion current may flow if the electrode materials have different electrode potentials. This happens mainly when the materials are different, but can also occur with electrodes made from the same material but different electrochemical properties caused by for example different fabrication processes. In neural stimulation, galvanic corrosion is especially important if the working and counter electrodes are connected for relatively long periods of time, usually more than several minutes, without a disturbing interrupt. Only then equilibrium is established in the system and the galvanic corrosion current becomes measurable.

If the stimulation frequency is so low that the distance between the stimulation pulses may extend as long as several minutes or longer and the stimulation electrodes are kept at the same potential as the counter electrode during this time, the galvanic corrosion current between the working and the counter electrodes must be measured and evaluated. The potentiostats do this by connecting the two electrodes together and measuring the current flowing. Enough time must be given to the system so that it becomes stable.

Galvanic corrosion measurement with the three different counter electrode materials was accomplished here. The resulting current curves for 200 points measured over 200 s are illustrated in Fig. 7.3.

As is seen in the figure, TiN counter electrode exhibits the highest average galvanic corrosion current. The average galvanic corrosion current is positive for TiN, i.e. it flows from the working into the counter electrode. Although in case of iridium this net current causes merely a slow oxidation of the iridium electrodes which is not harmful in this especial case, such a positive galvanic corrosion must be avoided in general, because it means stimulation electrode oxidization or metal dissolution. Despite consisting from the same material as the stimulation electrodes, the iridium counter electrode also does not feature a zero galvanic corrosion current, while gold is again the best material here exhibiting a nearly zero average current.

Reference

1. Mandel Y, Goetz G, Lavinsky D, Huie P, Mathieson K, Wang L, Kamins T, Galambos L, Manivanh R, Harris J, Palanker D (2013) Cortical responses elicited by photovoltaic subretinal prostheses exhibit similarities to visually evoked potentials. Nature Communications 4, DOI 10. 1038/ncomms2980

Chapter 8
Electrode Modeling for Titanium Nitride, Iridium and Iridium Oxide Microelectrodes

As stated before, electrodes are not standard linear electrical elements. Electrode properties depend on the electrode potential. Especially, in stimulation electrodes, the electrode potential fluctuates over a relatively wide range, thus enhancing the nonlinear characteristics of the electrode-electrolyte interface. However, an approximate electrical model can be helpful in designing the interface circuits to the electrodes, like signal recording or driver circuits. As explained in Chap. 5, impedance spectroscopy is one of the methods to extract the electrode model. In the following this and other methods are explained through practical examples.

8.1 Titanium Nitride

There are different theoretical and experimental ways to determine the electrode model in an application. There are various formulas to calculate the electrode elements in the literature. As mentioned above, the spreading resistance R_s is the resistance felt by the current as it spreads out into the fluid from the electrode. The equation for the spreading resistance of a square electrode is [1]:

$$R_s = \frac{\rho \cdot ln(4)}{\pi \cdot L}$$

where ρ is the resistivity of the solution (which is $64\,\Omega\,cm$ for the phosphate buffered saline used here) and L is the side length of the electrode. R_s depends only on the geometric surface area and not on the real surface area. It should also be noted that this equation assumes an infinitely large counter electrode. As an example the spreading resistance corresponding to the square electrodes having a side of $50\,\mu m$ used here (see Chap. 5) has a theoretical value of about $5.7\,k\Omega$.

© The Author(s) 2015
N. Pour Aryan et al., *Stimulation and Recording Electrodes for Neural Prostheses*,
SpringerBriefs in Electrical and Computer Engineering 78,
DOI 10.1007/978-3-319-10052-4_8

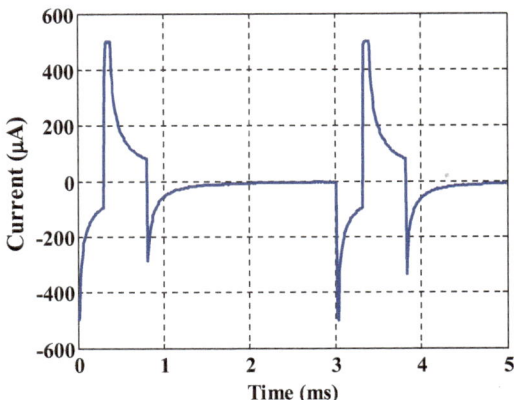

Fig. 8.1 Electrodes current in response to a ±1 V biphasic square voltage on 16 electrodes. Current measurement range was limited to ±500 μA

Calculating the interface capacitance C_I is more complicated. The interface capacitance is the total series capacitance of the surface Helmholtz capacitance and the so called Gouy-Chapman capacitance, corresponding to the diffuse area of space charge that follows the Helmholtz layer and neutralizes that amount of charge that is not immobilized directly on the metal surface [4]. A detailed calculation procedure for the interface capacitance of platinum, platinum black and titanium nitride as electrode materials is explained in [1].

Determining C_I is also possible through experiments. In Fig. 8.1 the resulting electrode current in response to a ±1 V biphasic square voltage is measured. Considering the simple electrode model of a resistor and a capacitor in series (Fig. 2.1b), the interface capacitor is calculated from the time constant of the exponential current decay (220 μs) and the above calculated R_s. The current measurement resistor of 470 Ω was taken into account. The nonlinear dependence of the titanium nitride interface capacitance on electrode voltage amplitude [5] was neglected. Here 16 neighboring electrodes each having an area of 50 × 50 μm where driven and measured in parallel. The total resistance contributing to the time constant is:

$$R_{Total} = \frac{R_s}{16} + R_{Meas.} = 830\ \Omega$$

Therefore, the resulting C_I per electrode is about 17 nF.

8.2 Iridium

Iridium electrode models have been seldom investigated in the literature. In this section modeling of iridium electrodes is studied.

As stated before, another method to experimentally determine the electrode model is to perform impedance spectroscopy by a potentiostat and curve fit the resulting diagrams through a curve-fitting software like ZView 2 (©2005 Scribner Associates, Inc.) to get the model which fits best the impedance spectrum measured. This approach was used to extract the electrode model of the disk iridium electrodes on a microelectrode array (MEA) as shown in Fig. 8.2. These electrodes could be accessed individually and had a diameter of 30 μm each. As mentioned before,

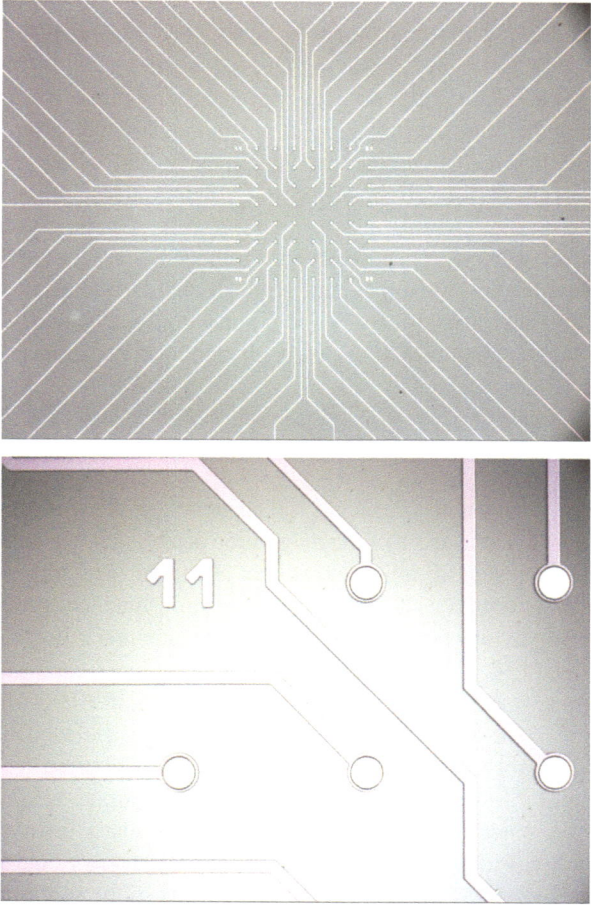

Fig. 8.2 Circular iridium electrodes used for impedance spectroscopy and electrode model extraction in this study. *Upper picture* shows the surface of a whole MEA, *lower picture* illustrates several disc electrodes zoomed on

two MEAs of this kind were available for the experiments labeled MEA 1 and MEA 2. In addition to ZView 2, Microsoft Excel was also used for data processing. For importing and processing data many macros (small programs) written in the programming language "Visual Basic for Applications" (VBA) which is a part of Microsoft Office were implemented.

Each MEA has 60 electrodes which were immersed in PBS. Impedance spectra of the electrodes for the frequency range of 1 Hz to 50 kHz were measured and are shown in Fig. 8.3. The colorful curves belong to MEA 1 and the pale ones belong to MEA 2. About 80 % of the measured amplitude spectra are similar and form a bundle of quasi-lines with falling magnitude versus frequency. The two lowest curves correspond to two macroelectrodes with the area of about 7 mm^2 each. Both have lower amplitude values due to their corresponding higher electrode-electrolyte interface capacitances. Both show a plateau at higher frequencies corresponding to the solution spreading resistance. The remaining electrodes are outliers whose spectra deviated a lot from the majority. Dirt was observed on some of these electrodes. In the following these outliers are ignored. In Fig. 8.3 the bottom graph contains the phase responses of the electrodes cleaned from the outliers. The microelectrodes have on average a constant phase of about $-70°$ over the frequency. This behavior together with the linearly falling impedance amplitude results in an electrode model consisting only of a constant phase element Z_{CPE} (or simply CPE).

Z_{CPE} is a measure of the non-faradaic impedance arising from the interface capacitance. It represents the impedance of the double layer capacitance in the presence of surface roughness effects. Z_{CPE} is the dominant factor in the interface impedance at high frequencies. Its value is given by the empirical relation [2]:

$$Z_{CPE}(\omega) = \frac{1}{T(j\omega)^n}$$

CPE is like a non-ideal capacitor (a capacitor with a constant phase shift lower than $90°$). T is a measure of the magnitude of Z_{CPE}. n is a constant parameter ($0 \leq n \leq 1$) representing inhomogeneities in the surface and ω is the angular frequency. In the case of $n = 1$, Z_{CPE} equals a pure capacitor corresponding to the electrode-electrolyte interface capacitance. The parameters n and T depend on the electrode material [3].

The average extracted CPE parameters of MEA 1 and MEA 2 microelectrodes are displayed in Table 8.1. In order to evaluate the interface capacitance in nF, the values for a capacitor used instead of the CPE as a model were also extracted and are included in Table 8.1. The capacitor is not as accurate as CPE in this case. A spreading resistance cannot be calculated for the microelectrodes because the impedance amplitude continues to fall linearly for higher frequencies and the phase remains a constant $-70°$. The quasi-RC time constant of the spreading resistance in series with the CPE is too small to be identified in this frequency range (Fig. 8.4).

For DC voltages ≥ 0.5 V a new phenomenon is visible in the impedance spectrum. The spectrum curve saturates for values below 25 Hz (Fig. 8.5). Due to the high

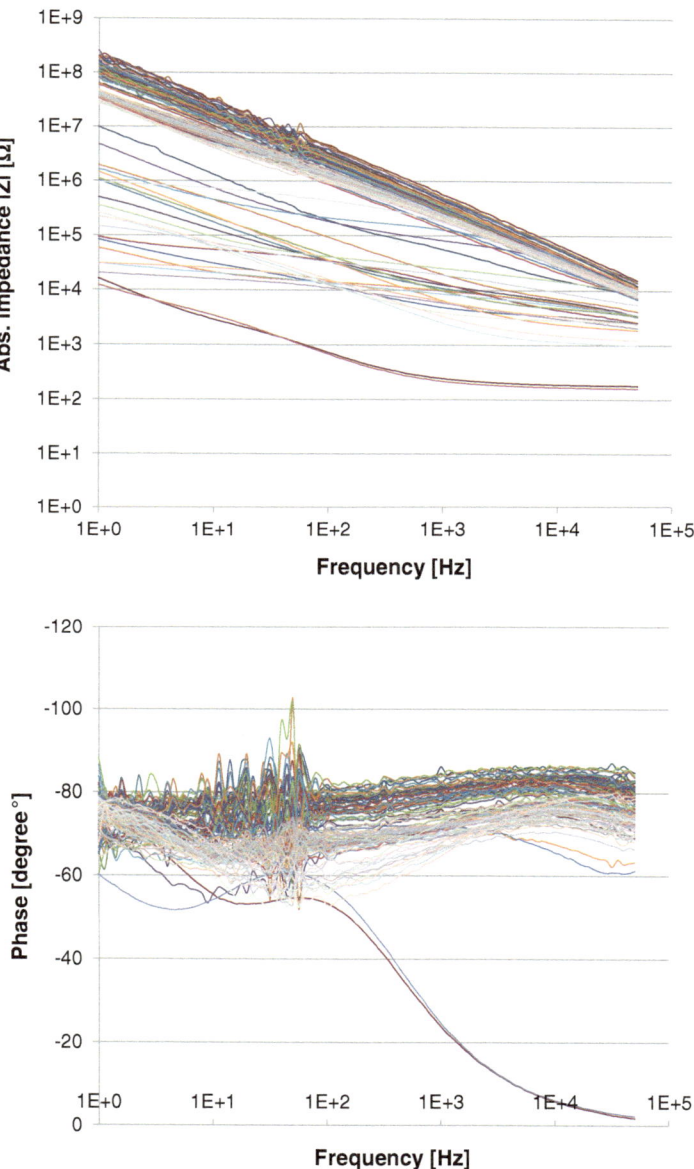

Fig. 8.3 *Above*: Impedance amplitude versus frequency of 120 electrodes of MEA 1 and MEA 2, *below*: Phase response of the electrodes with the outliers being removed

electrode voltage the faradaic resistance (R_{FW} in Fig. 3.2) becomes low enough to affect the impedance spectrum. By extrapolating the curve for lower frequencies an R_{FW} of several Megaohms can be estimated with this bias voltage. The existence of R_{FW} indicates the presence of some redox reactions on the electrode surface.

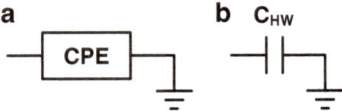

Fig. 8.4 Electrode model for the iridium electrodes composed only of (a) a single constant phase element or (b) a single capacitor

Table 8.1 CPE and capacitor (C_{HW}) values of the one-element models of Fig. 8.4 for the iridium electrodes

MEA 1	$T\ (\mathrm{F\,s}^{n-1})$	n	C_{HW} (nF)
Single element model	1.66E−9	0.868	0.59
MEA 2			
Single element model	5.89E−9	0.774	1.02

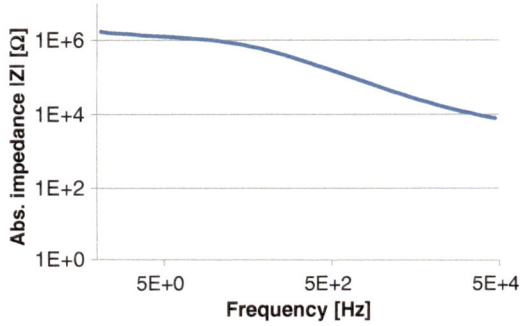

Fig. 8.5 Impedance amplitude spectrum for an iridium electrode with 0.5 V bias voltage (vs. OCP)

Because 0.5 V is still inside the water window, these reactions are reversible, although the occurrence of the corresponding reverse reactions requires a reduction of the bias voltage. A continuous 0.5 V DC voltage would hence damage the electrode if it lasts for a long time.

For the macroelectrodes, in addition to the CPE (or the capacitor), the spreading resistance R_S must be added to the model to account for the plateau observed in the higher frequency range. Also, as the area of the macroelectrode ($7\,\mathrm{mm}^2$) is not negligible compared to the counter electrode ($0.5\,\mathrm{cm}^2$), the impedance of the counter electrode cannot be neglected. The necessary model is the one shown in Fig. 2.1a. The resulting parameters extracted by ZView 2 are shown in Table 8.2. The macroelectrodes are coded as MEA1 MAE and MEA2 MAE. In the table two models are described for MEA1 MAE. One is the three-elements model of Fig. 2.1a and the other is the same except that the interface capacitor of the macroelectrode is replaced by a CPE. The latter shows a better agreement with the measured spectra. The relatively small value of R_S is due to the large area of the macroelectrode. The smaller interface capacitance was mapped to the macroelectrode because of its lower area.

Table 8.2 Parameters of the three-elements model of Fig. 2.1a corresponding to the iridium macroelectrodes extracted by ZView 2

MEA1 MAE	R_S	C_{HW}/T, n	C_{HC}
Three-elements model	197.8 Ω	2.6752 μF	8.644 μF
MEA1 MAE			
Three-elements model	160 Ω	2.40 E−5 (F s^{n-1}), 0.67	10.7 μF
including CPE			

C_{HW} and C_{HC} are the macroelectrode and the counter electrode interface capacitances, respectively

8.3   Iridium Electrode Activation and the Resulting Electrode Model

Figure 8.6 shows the average impedance spectra of the ten MEA 1 electrodes for different activation levels. As activation continues and the oxide layer on the electrodes builds up, the electrode capacitance increases and the electrode impedance decreases specially for lower frequencies. The impedance decrease from 400 cycles level to 500 cycles level is relatively small. Impedance decrease versus activation level was also observed for MEA 2 which was activated by totally 1,500 cycles. Also for MEA 2 impedance fall was relatively small for activation beyond 300 cycles.

With the increase in the quasi-RC time constant of the series connection of R_S and CPE, its value can be recognized by the spectra of higher activation levels. Now R_S can be determined to be 10.6 kΩ from the diagram corresponding to 500 activation cycles, where the impedance saturates at higher frequencies. As R_s depends only on electrode geometry and solution resistivity, the same value is also valid for not activated electrodes, where because of the low quasi-RC time constant it could not be determined previously. So the above mentioned one-element model consisting only of a CPE (or capacitor) can be corrected by adding a series R_S resistance.

The spreading resistance of a disc electrode with a diameter d is calculated by [1]:

$$R_S = \frac{\rho}{2d}$$

from which a resistivity of 64 Ω cm is obtained for the PBS solution used here. Using the simple electrode model of Fig. 2.1a and $R_S = 10.6$ kΩ the capacitor values are determined by ZView 2 and included in Table 8.3. Agreement to the model was higher for higher activation levels. Substituting the capacitor by a CPE improved the overall agreement. The extracted values for CPE are also shown in Table 8.3. According to the table, the double layer capacitance increases more than 100 times during the activation period. For MEA 1 electrodes, the capacitance per electrode increases from 0.6 to 89.5 nF after 500 activation cycles. In MEA 2, the

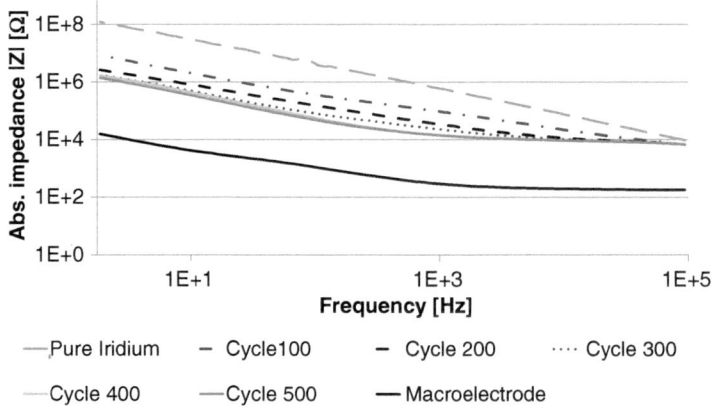

—Pure Iridium   − Cycle100   − Cycle 200   ···· Cycle 300

—Cycle 400   —Cycle 500   — Macroelectrode

Fig. 8.6 Average impedance amplitude spectra of MEA 1 electrodes for different activation levels. The macroelectrode was not activated

Table 8.3 Parameters of the series RC model and the quasi-RC model in which the capacitor is replaced by CPE; R_S was set to 10.6 kΩ

MEA 1 cycles	T (nF s^{n-1})/ C_{HW} (nF)	n	MEA 2 cycles	T (nF s^{n-1})/ C_{HW} (nF)	n
0	1.7/0.6	0.868	0	6.0/1.0	0.776
100	46.4/7.5	0.705	–	–	–
200	98.3/24.0	0.731	200	100.3/40.2	0.796
300	154.0/50.6	0.751	300	135.0/55.0	0.784
400	118.8/70.1	0.860	500	141.3/67.7	0.826
500	158.4/89.5	0.845	1,500	246.8/152.8	0.854

capacitance per electrode increases from 1.0 to 67.7 nF after 500 and to 152.8 nF after 1,500 activation cycles.

From Tables 8.3 and 6.3 it is seen that through activation, the electrode-electrolyte interface capacitance increases more than 100 times while the charge injection capacity increases only about 10 times. Because of the intrinsic delays present in the topography of the electrode surface structures, like the pores RC delays as was illustrated in Fig. 1.3, the whole interface capacitance ($\propto$ electrochemical surface area (ESA)) is not accessible at higher activation levels for the applied biphasic voltage signals. Other factors which reduce the accessible charge injection capacity for fast signals are the limited diffusion rates of the charge carriers in the solution [5] and the kinetics of the reactions contributing to the "pseudo capacitive charge injection mechanisms" explained in Sect. 6.2.1.

References

1. Franks W, Schenker I, Schmutz P, Hierlemann A (2005) Impedance characterization and modeling of electrodes for biomedical applications. Biomedical Engineering, IEEE Transactions on 52(7):1295–1302, DOI 10.1109/TBME.2005.847523
2. McAdams ET, Lackermeier A, McLaughlin JA, Macken D, Jossinet J (1995) The linear and non-linear electrical properties of the electrode-electrolyte interface. Biosensors and Bioelectronics 10(1–2):67–74, URL http://www.sciencedirect.com/science/article/pii/095656639596795Z
3. Poppendieck W (2010) Untersuchungen zum Einsatz neuer Elektrodenmaterialien: Und deren Evaluation als Reiz- und Ableitelektrode. Südwestdeutscher Verlag, URL http://books.google.de/books?id=Z1xnRwAACAAJ
4. Stieglitz T (2004) Materials for stimulation and recording. Tech. rep., Neural Prosthetics Group, Fraunhofer Institute for Biomedical Engineering
5. Weiland JD, Anderson DJ, Humayun MS (2002) In vitro electrical properties for iridium oxide versus titanium nitride stimulating electrodes. Biomedical Engineering, IEEE Transactions on 49(12):1574–1579, DOI 10.1109/TBME.2002.805487

Chapter 9
Summary

In this book, after investigating the principal electrochemical theories concerning the electrodes and the measurement methods like cyclic voltammetry and impedance spectroscopy, the chemistry and the concept behind the water window was explained. It was also shown how charge balance is necessary to acquire a long electrode lifetime.

We saw how the electrode geometry affects the electrode stability and endurance and introduced methods to enhance lifetime through a better geometrical design. As it was further explained, in case of electrostimulation, signal waveforms must also lack high frequency components if longer operation durations are required.

In this study, beside using standard measurement devices like potentiostat, new hardware was designed and implemented in order to investigate microelectrodes. The electrode materials under investigation were iridium, iridium oxide and titanium nitride. It was shown that these can provide more charge injection capacity compared to the traditionally used platinum. Other alternatives like conducting polymers are also studied worldwide and may come to practical applications soon.

A new topic covered here is the effect of the counter electrode material on the faradaic reactions and galvanic corrosion in a two electrode monopolar stimulation system. It was explained how selecting a proper material for the counter electrode can enhance the electrode lifetime.

In the following last chapter, electrical models were extracted for the microelectrodes under investigation using impedance spectroscopy and current measurement while applying biphasic square voltages on the electrodes.

© The Author(s) 2015   81
N. Pour Aryan et al., *Stimulation and Recording Electrodes for Neural Prostheses*,
SpringerBriefs in Electrical and Computer Engineering 78,
DOI 10.1007/978-3-319-10052-4_9